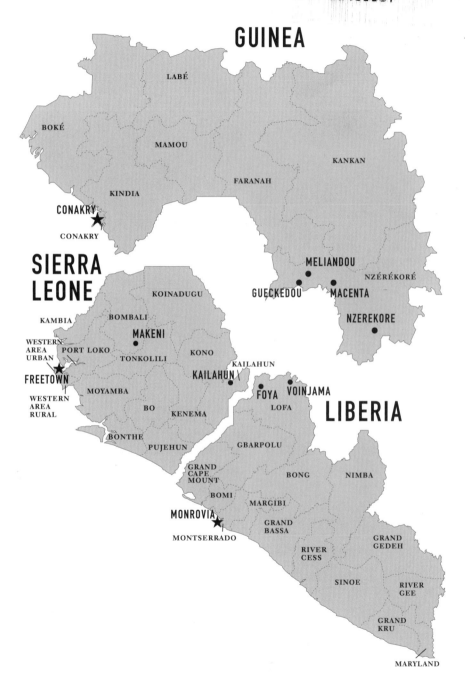

GUINEA

LABÉ

BOKÉ

MAMOU

KANKAN

FARANAH

KINDIA

CONAKRY

CONAKRY

SIERRA
LEONE

KOINADUGU

MELIANDOU

NZÉRÉKORÉ

GUECKEDOU

MACENTA

KAMBIA

BOMBALI

MAKENI

NZEREKORE

WESTERN
AREA
URBAN

PORT LOKO

TONKOLILI

KONO

KAILAHUN

FREETOWN

KAILAHUN

MOYAMBA

FOYA

VOINJAMA

WESTERN
AREA
RURAL

BO

KENEMA

LOFA

LIBERIA

BONTHE

PUJEHUN

GBARPOLU

GRAND
CAPE
MOUNT

BONG

NIMBA

BOMI

MARGIBI

MONROVIA

GRAND
BASSA

MONTSERRADO

RIVER
CESS

GRAND
GEDEH

SINOE

RIVER
GEE

GRAND
KRU

MARYLAND

EPIDEMIC

EPIDEMIC

Ebola and the Global Race to Prevent the Next Killer Outbreak

REID WILSON

BROOKINGS INSTITUTION PRESS

Washington, D.C.

The Brookings Institution is a private nonprofit organization devoted to research, education, and publication on important issues of domestic and foreign policy. Its principal purpose is to bring the highest quality independent research and analysis to bear on current and emerging policy problems. Interpretations or conclusions in Brookings publications should be understood to be solely those of the authors.

Library of Congress Cataloging-in-Publication data are available.
ISBN 978-0-8157-3135-1 (cloth : alk. paper)
ISBN 978-0-8157-3136-8 (ebook)

9 8 7 6 5 4 3 2 1

Typeset in Electra

Composition by Westchester Publishing Services

For Veronica and Max
my two inspirations

Contents

Cast of Characters

In West Africa

Ellen Johnson Sirleaf · President of Liberia

Alpha Conde · President of Guinea

Ernest Bai Koroma · President of Sierra Leone

Tolbert Nyenswah · Assistant minister of health, Liberia; head of Incident Management System

Tamba Boima · Director, Community Health Services Division, Ministry of Health, Liberia

Mosaka Fallah · Epidemiologist and immunologist

Hans Rosling · International health expert, Karolinska Institute

Sheik Umar Khan · Head of Lassa Fever Program, Kenema Government Hospital

Robert Garry · Professor of Microbiology and Immunology, Tulane University

Piet deVries · Country director for Liberia, Global Communities

Brett Sedgewick · Director of development services, Global Communities

George Woryonwon · Global Communities

David Robinson · Senior adviser for operations, World Vision International

Craig Spencer · Médecins Sans Frontières (Doctors Without Borders)

Kent Brantly · Samaritan's Purse

Nancy Writebol · Serving in Mission

David Blackley · Epidemiologist, U.S. Centers for Disease Control and Prevention

Barry Fields · Microbiologist, U.S. Centers for Disease Control and Prevention

Peter Kilmarx · Ebola response team leader, U.S. Centers for Disease Control and Prevention, Sierra Leone; deputy team leader, U.S. Centers for Disease Control and Prevention, Guinea

Kim Lindblade · Epidemiologist, U.S. Centers for Disease Control and Prevention

Joe Woodring   Senior medical officer, National Center for Health Statistics, U.S. Centers for Disease Control and Prevention

Dan Martin   Public health adviser, U.S. Centers for Disease Control and Prevention

Leisha Nolen   Epidemic Intelligence Service, U.S. Centers for Disease Control and Prevention

Deborah Malac   U.S. ambassador to Liberia

Darryl Williams   Major general, commander, United States Army Africa

Gary Volesky   Major general, commander, 101st Airborne Division

Ross Lightsey   Lieutenant colonel, 101st Airborne Division

Tony Costello   Major, 36th Engineer Brigade

Jeff Kugelman   Captain, U.S. Army Medical Research Institute for Infectious Diseases

Michael Schmoyer   Captain, U.S. Public Health Service

Fabian Leendertz   Epidemiologist, Robert Koch Institute

In Atlanta

Tom Frieden   Director, U.S. Centers for Disease Control and Prevention

Charlie Stokes   President and chief executive officer, U.S. Centers for Disease Control and Prevention Foundation

At the U.S. Army Medical Research Institute for Infectious Diseases, Fort Detrick, Maryland

John Dye   Chief of Viral Immunology

Brian Gentile   Colonel, director of administration

David Norwood   Chief of Diagnostic Systems Division

Randy Schoepp   Virologist

Travis Warren   Principal investigator, Division of Molecular and Translational Sciences

In Geneva

Margaret Chan   Director-general, World Health Organization

Christopher Dye   Director of strategy, Office of the Director-General, World Health Organization

Gregory Hartl   Spokesman, World Health Organization

In Miami

Julio Frenk   President, University of Miami; member, World Health Organization Ebola Interim Assessment Panel

Preface

THE OUTBREAK OF EBOLA Virus Disease began in 2013 in a small town in rural Guinea. From there, it spread to Liberia, then Sierra Leone, then across borders into Nigeria, Mali, Europe, and the United States. In the end, more than 28,000 people were infected, and 11,325 lost their lives. Dozens of organizations fought the disease, from global organizations like the United Nations and governments like that of the United States to nongovernmental groups like Médecins Sans Frontières, the Red Crescent/ Red Cross, and Global Communities. Together, thousands of responders poured into West Africa to aid the thousands more Guineans, Liberians, and Sierra Leoneans who took it upon themselves to save their own countries.

All those who helped save lives deserve recognition, but it is not possible to tell their stories in one place. Instead, my aim is to relate the broader story of the global response to the outbreak, with a special focus on the United States government's work to combat Ebola, while shining a spotlight on the weak state of global health preparedness. While this volume's goal is to be as comprehensive as possible, I am aware, regretfully, that many heroes of that period will be left out.

Dozens of sources were interviewed for this work over hundreds of hours, beginning even before the outbreak formally ended. The vast majority of those sources spoke on the record. In the few instances where those sources asked for anonymity to discuss sensitive topics, I have sought to provide as much contextual information about their identities as those sources would allow.

EPIDEMIC

Introduction

TOM FRIEDEN FELT THE sweat dripping down his face in the oppressive humidity of equatorial Africa. Dressed in head-to-toe protective gear, peering through the plastic face mask, he struggled to come to terms with the scene of desperation as he walked through a hospital ward in the slums of Monrovia, Liberia's capital. All around him, he gazed into the faces of the dying, dozens of patients suffering from a terrifying virus that melted their bodies from the inside.

As Frieden walked the aisles, he came to a fourteen-year-old boy sitting on a rickety wooden chair. The young man was barely conscious, a state that so often accompanies the end stages of this particular pathogen. It was clear he had just days, maybe only hours, to live. A bottle of liquid, rehydration solution, sat next to the boy. Frieden begged him to drink as much as he could.

A few beds down the row, Frieden met a young woman who had lived through her ordeal with the virus. She had cared for her husband when he got sick, cared for his body when he died, and she had survived the worst hell on earth after she came down with the virus herself. But the woman had a vacant stare that the lone doctor on the ward, Armand Sprecher, told Frieden had become a common trait among those who survived. It was not clear to doctors and scientists studying this deadly disease whether the stare was from shock, from fluid build-up that caused brain swelling, or from something else entirely. In previous outbreaks, so few people had actually survived that no one had a chance to study the aftereffects. "We see this in survivors and we don't know what it is," Sprecher told Frieden.

Amid the heat, the humidity, the moans of human suffering, Frieden saw another woman lying facedown on her cot. He was struck by her hair, woven into beautiful braids that must have taken hours of careful, loving work. Then Frieden noticed the flies on the woman's legs. He realized she had died during the night, but her body had not yet been moved. A man next to the dead woman complained that the body was a risk to the rest of the patients struggling to survive. Sprecher explained to the man that they needed four staffers to move a body. Patients were dying too fast for the few remaining staffers to cart them off. Throughout the ward, sixty corpses lay among the living and the dying, waiting to be transferred to a crematorium that was working overtime to burn infected bodies. There was no one to remove the bodies, no one to clean the mess of blood and vomit and diarrhea that coated beds and floors. So many were ill that Sprecher and his dwindling team of nurses did not have time to put IVs into the patients' arms.

Frieden and Sprecher are no strangers to human suffering. Sprecher works with Médecins Sans Frontières, known in the United States as Doctors Without Borders, where he spent a career fighting viruses in Uganda, Angola, and the Democratic Republic of the Congo before being deployed to Liberia. Frieden, the director of the Centers for Disease Control and Prevention in Atlanta, had responded to some of the deadliest disasters in the remotest parts of the world.

"I've worked in earthquakes, hurricanes, tornadoes. I've seen famine, I've worked in war zones," Frieden said later, recalling his visit to the hospital in Monrovia. "I've never seen anything like that. I mean, it was a scene out of Dante."

When Frieden returned to the United States a few days later, he called the White House, where he was patched through to President Obama. Frieden, agitated after a long transoceanic flight, told Obama what he had seen: the grisly makeshift hospital, three West African nations, already the poorest in the world, decimated by a virus that had claimed the lives of hundreds of health care workers and now left adrift without the help they so desperately needed to fight back. The World Health Organization, ostensibly the agency that was supposed to head the response, was so woefully overmatched for the task, Frieden told Obama, that a global spread of a deadly virus was possible, if not probable. The American government was the only actor with the capacity to stop what could become a global pandemic of an incurable disease.

The virus that raged from remote forest villages to crowded slums of major capitals is one of the most deadly pathogens ever discovered; in previous outbreaks, nine out of every ten people infected had died, often in gruesome ways. It is named for a small subtributary of the mighty Congo River, near the site where four decades ago villagers came down with a hemorrhagic fever that terrified the first Westerners to see it. That small subtributary is called the Ebola River.

By the time Frieden returned to the United States after his eye-opening trip, five months had passed since the World Health Organization had confirmed the presence of the Ebola virus in Guinea. Scientists would later discover it had actually been about eight months since the first victim, known in epidemiological parlance as Patient Zero, fell ill. Just weeks after Patient Zero died, Ebola had spread across the border to Liberia. After a brief moment of cautious optimism that the disease was under control, it appeared in Sierra Leone. Like a horrible feedback loop, the virus was now amplifying itself, and those few epidemiologists brave enough to put themselves in harm's way were beginning to warn that the situation was spinning out of control.

In the forty years since scientists first identified the virus, Ebola had never reached a city of significant size. Now, Frieden and his counterparts in the global health community watched as Ebola reached three major cities at the same time—Conakry, Monrovia, and Freetown, capitals with populations reaching a million people packed tightly into poor and crowded slums. Those slums were ideal incubators for the highly contagious virus. More worrisome, that meant the virus had, for the first time in recorded history, reached cities served by daily direct flights to Europe and the Middle East. All the epidemic needed to become a pandemic was for the right person to buy a plane ticket.

Two realizations hit Frieden and his counterparts, Anthony Fauci, head of the National Institute of Allergy and Infectious Diseases, and Rajiv Shah, the director of the U.S. Agency for International Development. The first was that a combination of factors—dense populations and crushing poverty in massive slums, and the cultural funerary traditions that put family members in close contact with their deceased relatives—meant this outbreak, already the worst in recorded history, was unlike any they had ever seen. The second was that the global health community was woefully unprepared to respond and incapable of marshaling the resources necessary to stop it.

In West Africa alone, thousands, if not hundreds of thousands, of lives were at stake. Globally, millions could be at risk.

The days of an isolated outbreak of a contagious disease are over. Every city of any size, in the modern globalized world, is one connection away from Washington or New York or Beijing or Jakarta. Today's outbreak in West Africa, if left unchecked, is tomorrow's global pandemic. Someone had to fight Ebola in West Africa, to prevent a global outbreak that could threaten millions of lives.

Every fire starts with a spark. Every spark, under the right circumstances, can become a conflagration burning out of control, consuming everything within its path—a house, a forest, a people, a country.

The spark that landed in the unique tinderbox of West Africa was made of a few strands of ribonucleic acid, a set of genetic code that, when it comes into contact with human cells, begins rapidly multiplying, searching voraciously for anything that can fuel its growth. The impacts on the human body can be horrifying to witness: bleeding, vomiting, diarrhea, a slow, painful, and violent death. All the while, the small flame is searching for its next host, and the fire spreads.

The Ebola outbreak that killed 11,325 people in West Africa over more than a year and a half was unlike any other epidemic the global health community had seen. Many of the dozens of people interviewed for this book use the same phrase to describe the conditions that contributed to its appearance and spread: the perfect storm.

The circumstances were seemingly tailor-made for a humanitarian disaster of epic proportions: the disease showed up in an area where it had never before appeared, where conditions for its rapid spread were aided by a combination of ancient traditions and modern transportation, all colliding in three desperately poor countries where the medical infrastructure was already teetering on the brink of collapse.

At the same time, the outbreak exposed a woefully inadequate global response network that was ostensibly supposed to find and fight deadly pathogens. After decades of bloat, international organizations had become so overburdened by bureaucracy and corruption that they could not possibly handle a disease of Ebola's magnitude.

The story of the Ebola outbreak in West Africa is one of incredible lows and incredible highs, of terrible luck and unbelievably good fortunes. It is a story of countries consumed by terror, of politicians taking advantage of fear, and of heroes who ran toward the unfolding disaster, many of whom lost their own lives. It is a story of the past, with deep roots in colonial history, and of the future, with ramifications for the next time the world faces a deadly pathogen. And it is a story of dramatic innovation across the globe—ingenuity and creativity that saved tens of thousands, maybe hundreds of thousands of lives.

"When this is a movie," said Gayle Smith, who oversaw the American response at the National Security Council, "people will say you overdid it."

Most of all, it is a story of determination and hope—determination by thousands of West Africans and their friends around the world to save their countries, and hope that the combination of new approaches that helped stop this disaster in its tracks can do the same next time, before thousands of lives are lost.

And that next time is coming. The global population is expanding, moving closer and closer to previously untouched wilderness where viruses like Ebola lurk, at the same time the world is becoming ever more connected. The question is not whether another virus will attack humanity, it is whether someone infected will be able to get on a transcontinental flight when that attack happens—and whether the countries affected will respond quickly enough.

The next sparks are out there, looking for fuel. This is the story of one of the greatest threats the medical world has ever faced, and the lessons it learned that could prevent the next threat from becoming an uncontrollable global inferno.

Our story begins in the remote hills of West Africa, where peace had finally taken hold after more than a decade of war. The next war began with a two-year-old child.

ONE

Emile

BETWEEN THE LOW-LYING MOUNTAINS of southwestern Guinea, the small village of Meliandou sits atop a remote and barren hillside, overlooking coffee plantations and rice paddies. Residents live in thirty-one cinder-block homes with makeshift shutters, some painted green, some topped with corrugated tin roofs, separated by narrow unpaved alleys, connected by laundry lines on which shirts and sheets dry under the hot African sun. They are connected to the outside world by a single, bumpy red dirt road, and a lone bridge that is so rickety that the few visitors who venture so far out into the hills tend to test it before rolling their cars over the wood planks. Villagers commute by car and bus to nearby towns to sell spinach, corn, and bananas. In a region of remote outposts of human existence, separated by miles of track through the jungle, Meliandou stands out. It is so isolated that the only working well in the area is across the bridge. Its name, in the local Kissi language, means "this is as far as we go."

Meliandou sits in the most insular part of the three countries that make up the southwest coast of West Africa. The village is just a few miles from where those three countries—Guinea, Sierra Leone, and Liberia—meet at a single point.

The children of Meliandou, far up in the Guinean mountains, contented themselves by playing in the lush nature that surrounded them. A hollow tree on the edge of the village was particularly appealing. It was home to a colony of fruit bats; if the kids timed their swipes just right, they could sometimes catch a bat and grill it over a small fire, adding a little protein to their diets.

The tree sat at the edge of the forest, through a field of waist-high grass about fifty meters from Emile Ouamouno's home, on a path villagers used to access a nearby stream.[1] One day in late November or early December 2013, the two-year-old wandered near the tree, perhaps as his mother worked nearby, just to play. Maybe a bat bit Emile. Maybe he touched some guano, then touched his eye. Whatever happened, in a single moment, a microscopic particle, a fraction of the size of a human blood cell, entered Emile's body. It attached itself to one of his cells, and a sequence of ribonucleic acid, RNA, began replicating. It made dozens of copies of itself, then hundreds, then millions.

Days later, Emile developed a fever. He began vomiting. There was blood in his stool. His mother could do nothing but care for her son as he deteriorated, quickly, in her arms. On December 6, not even three years after he was born, Emile died. Scientists from the World Health Organization would later conclude Emile had been the first victim of that microscopic particle called Ebola.[2] Today, his body lies beneath an unmarked grave, identified only by the stones placed atop it. Villagers, afraid of the silent and invisible killer unleashed in their midst, burned the tree that housed the bats.

How the Ebola virus actually spreads from animal hosts to humans— a process known as zoonosis—is not exactly clear to scientists. Before it reaches a human body, the virus lives within another species peacefully, without causing symptoms. That other species that houses a virus is called the reservoir host, and just about any species can be a reservoir host for something: fleas on rats carried the bubonic plague, mice carry hantavirus, mosquitoes carry the Zika virus and chikungunya, two diseases currently racing across the planet. But when it comes to Ebola, scientists still do not know with complete certainty what animal carries the virus when it is not infecting humans. The reservoir host is probably a bat, though no one can say for sure exactly which species of bat is at fault. Investigators who visited

Meliandou after the fact captured eighty-eight bats, most of them Angolan free-tailed bats, the same species that lived in the hollowed out tree; none showed signs of the virus.

But how Ebola spreads from human to human is abundantly clear: billions of virus particles infest every drop of an infected victim's bodily fluid. The slightest contact can lead to infection. When another person touches bodily fluid, the virus spreads, either through tiny abrasions in the skin or mucus membranes, like the eye or mouth. And as the virus spreads through one host, it creates the conditions for its own leap to another host. As Ebola takes hold in a body, that person becomes more and more contagious; at the moment of death, a body is at its most contagious, like a land mine ready to explode, organic shrapnel endangering anyone within reach.

As Emile worsened, he became more and more of a risk to those around him. He died in his grandmother's house, across the village from the home where he had spent his short life, where he had shared a bed with his pregnant mother. She became ill just days later; she gave birth to a stillborn baby a few days after that, and within a week of her son, she too was dead. Emile's three-year-old sister broke out in a fever on Christmas Day. She died four days later.

It did not take long for Emile's grandmother to feel sick, too. She did not trust the shaman who had tried traditional healing practices, with no effect, on her daughter and grandchildren, so she traveled to Gueckedou, the closest city of any size—home to 80,000 residents—which sits right at the border with Liberia and Sierra Leone. There, the grandmother stayed with a friend, a nurse who worked in the city's hospital. Days of treatment did not reverse her symptoms, so she returned to Meliandou, where she became the fourth victim.

Cholera and other diseases killed frequently in Meliandou. But no one in the village had any idea what was ravaging Emile's family. Some believed the family was cursed by the gods, or by someone they had wronged. Some believed the entire village was cursed.

The Ebola virus disease has infected humans in dozens of towns and villages across Africa since it was first discovered in 1976. Many of those outbreaks come and go, raging and burning themselves out in remote corners of jungle so fast that those who are infected do not have the chance to seek medical treatment in a larger community, where the virus could jump to a new host. So, too, might the outbreak in Meliandou have ended, once the first victims passed away.

But while Meliandou may be remote, it is tied tightly enough to neighboring villages, through generations of tribal relations, that people nearby knew Emile's grandmother. Hundreds of mourners came to her funeral. Ritual demands that those mourners prepare the body for burial, touching her infected body and washing her for the afterlife. The funeral offered the virus its best opportunity to leave Meliandou. It leapt to the grandmother's sister, who took it with her to her village, Dawa. She died January 26, four weeks after her sister; a day earlier, another Dawa villager came down with a fever and bleeding.

Jean Claude Kpoghomou, a doctor in another small village called Tekolo, was nervous. He had heard about the deaths in Meliandou, caused by a strange fever that looked to him like cholera. Diseases like cholera, malaria, and dysentery were common in West Africa, deadly but treatable, more cause for concern than panic. Two years before, a major cholera outbreak had claimed lives in the Forest Region, and Kpoghomou worried it might be back. On January 24, he called a superior to report that cholera had returned. That superior called his own boss at a health office in Gueckedou, who in turn called a regional health director in Nzerekore. The director alerted Guinea's Ministry of Health in Conakry.[3] It was their first hint that something was wrong. A small team of Guinean and World Health Organization (WHO) officials visited Meliandou to investigate. They too believed they were looking at cholera. The idea that they might be facing Ebola, the deadliest virus known to mankind, never occurred to them. As far as anyone knew, Ebola was a disease of Central African countries like Uganda and the Democratic Republic of the Congo. It had never been found in Guinea or anywhere close to Guinea.

"Part of the difficulty [in identifying the Ebola virus] was that the likely suspected cause of the outbreak was cholera," Chris Dye, WHO's director of Strategy, Policy and Information recalled later. "If you go into the investigation with the view that you're looking for a bacterial infection like cholera, you very well may miss a virus like Ebola."

At the same time, the virus took another route out of Meliandou, when the nurse who had hosted Emile's grandmother became sick. The nurse traveled to Macenta, another town of almost 90,000 people, to see a friend who was a doctor. The doctor lived in a small home with his son, who shared a room with the nurse for a single night. The next day, the nurse visited Macenta's hospital. In the waiting room, he collapsed and died.

Months later, in a report published in the *New England Journal of Medicine*, thirty-one scientists identified the nurse, clinically referred to as S14, or the fourteenth suspected case of Ebola, as the tinder that turned a small spark in a remote corner of Guinea's Forest Region into a roaring flame. In the six days between his first symptoms, on February 5, and his death, on February 10, he helped the disease travel through several districts in Gueckedou, then to Macenta.

The doctor who hosted the nurse was the next victim, and the virus's next potential path to a larger population. He was stunned at the nurse's death—and perhaps more shocked when he himself came down with a fever. The doctor alerted the regional health authorities in Nzerekore, the second time they were warned that some deadly disease was present. The doctor left Macenta for Conakry; had epidemiologists known the Ebola virus was traveling toward an impoverished city of a million people, panic would certainly have set in. But the virus's first effort to reach Conakry died, along with the doctor, somewhere along the bumpy dirt roads that lead through the rural counties. His body was taken to Kissidougou to be buried. Soon the first cases began to appear in Kissidougou.

The doctor's son, who had spent a night in the same room as the infected nurse, developed his own symptoms. So did a colleague of the doctor's who worked in the hospital's lab. Then a nurse and the doctor's two brothers. All five died.

Back in Gueckedou, Dr. Alexis Traore watched his hospital fill up fast with patients experiencing the same symptoms: vomiting and diarrhea. The vast majority did not recover. Traore was the first medical professional in Guinea to begin to suspect that they might not be dealing with another cholera epidemic. The patients he was seeing all had fevers, a symptom that does not occur with cholera.

But when the doctor ordered tests, his hypothesis appeared incorrect. Cholera is rampant in West Africa, and early treatment is essential to survival. Therefore, the tests on hand at the hospital in Gueckedou were designed to sound alarms at even the smallest hint of the disease. That allowed the earliest possible warning, to facilitate faster treatment. It also resulted in false positives. Tests on seven of the nine patients under Traore's care were positive for cholera.

The death of the doctor in Macenta and the spread of the mystery illness into Kissidougou shook the staff at the regional health office in Nzerekore. But by the time they reported the outbreaks to the Ministry of Health in Conakry, nearly thirty people had died in at least eight cities and towns. Finally, Guinean officials asked for help from the World Health Organization, based in Geneva. Those officials began at step one of any medical crisis: tracking those who had come into contact with the last known victim in an attempt to re-create the path of contagion. The process, one of the most elemental in the practice of epidemiology, is called contact tracing.

Within days, the tracing led the first WHO investigators from the nurse who died in Macenta to the outbreak at Traore's hospital in Gueckedou. It was the first hint that the two clusters were somehow connected. WHO officials began to suspect they were dealing with a hemorrhagic fever—though once again, they settled on the wrong answer: Lassa.

Lassa fever is better known and better understood than Ebola. It is endemic to West Africa, where it is transmitted from rats to humans. First detected by Western scientists in 1969, when two missionaries died in the town of Lassa, Nigeria, it infects between 100,000 and 300,000 people every year. Of those, about 5,000 die. Those who are lucky experience only a mild fever, a headache, and pronounced weakness as the virus runs its course. Those who are not so lucky—about one in five patients—experience vomiting, facial swelling, and even hearing loss. The most unlucky will die within two weeks of multiple organ failure.[4]

The Lassa diagnosis made sense, more sense than cholera. In some areas of Sierra Leone and Liberia, between 10 percent and 16 percent of all patients admitted to hospitals each year test positive for Lassa. When word reached Esther Sterk, an epidemiologist in Geneva with Médecins Sans Frontières (MSF)—known in the United States as Doctors Without Borders—on March 14 that a mysterious disease was killing people in the Forest Region of Guinea, she initially assumed Lassa had reared its head. She forwarded a report describing the symptoms to Michel Van Herp, MSF's top hemorrhagic fever epidemiologist.

But Van Herp, who had spent time on the ground in Africa responding to outbreaks of all kinds of nasty bugs, wondered if something else was killing Guinean villagers.

"It is definitely a hemorrhagic fever," Van Herp told his colleagues. "We must really take into consideration that it is worse than Lassa. I think it's Ebola."[5]

Van Herp had made the leap no one else in Geneva had: the virus that was beginning to spread in West Africa might be something altogether new for the region. No one in the area—not the medicine man in Meliandou, not the doctor in Macenta, not Traore in Gueckedou, not even Ministry of Health officials in Conakry—had ever seen Ebola before. Every previous outbreak had happened in Sudan, the Democratic Republic of the Congo, Gabon and Uganda. Those countries were 2,000 miles away from Guinea, a virtual world apart.

Around the same time, the same reports reached Dr. Pierre Formenty. Formenty is one of the world's top Ebola experts, a WHO epidemiologist who had spent two decades fighting the worst infectious diseases as they broke out in remote corners of the globe. That March he was in the Democratic Republic of the Congo at a three-day training session to teach medical professionals how to take blood samples from suspected Ebola patients. E-mails from colleagues at WHO, describing the symptoms in Guinea, said that transmission of the new disease had occurred after funerals, when the deceased were washed and buried according to local custom.

It is not possible, Formenty knew, to transmit Lassa fever after death. He ruled out Marburg, another hemorrhagic fever similar to Ebola, as the root cause of the outbreak. Marburg's reservoir host, the animal in which it rests until it finds a human carrier, is the Roussettus bat, which lives in colonies in caves, and most people infected by Marburg come into contact with the disease while mining those caves. The mining industry in Guinea is based on open-cut pits, which are not good habitats for large Roussettus colonies. Postmortem transmission of a hemorrhagic fever in an area ill-suited to Marburg suggested only one thing to Formenty: Ebola.[6]

A few days later, a team of WHO scientists and Ministry of Health officials traveled to the Forest Region from Conakry to trace contacts as far back as they could. The path led them, eventually, down that single unpaved road, into Meliandou. For the first time, they identified Emile as the initial victim.

As the WHO team traced contacts backward to Meliandou, they discovered other branches of the disease radiating out from the tiny village, across international lines. Two weeks earlier, on March 3, a thirty-seven-year-old woman named Sia Wanda Koniono had died after suffering symptoms identical to the others. Koniono had come from a village across the border in Sierra Leone. A second woman still in Sierra Leone, Koniono's daughter, had also taken ill. An in-law, Kumba Yaya, had just died in a hospital there.[7]

Another woman, Finda Tamba, had left Guinea when she fell ill, to seek treatment at a hospital in Foya-Borma in neighboring Liberia. As in Guinea, Liberian medical officials had no idea what Ebola was and no idea how to protect themselves. Tamba died on March 20. Her sister, Tewa Joseph, soon became ill.[8]

Faced with mounting evidence that a hemorrhagic fever was burning in remote rural corners of three countries, the international medical community mobilized. MSF, often the first nongovernmental organization to land in a danger zone, deployed three emergency teams, one from neighboring Sierra Leone, one from Geneva, and one from Brussels. The first team arrived on-site on March 18. They began collecting blood samples from victims of the outbreak. They wrapped the samples in three layers of protective materials designed to absorb any spills. Those samples left Guinea through Conakry on March 21, in the cargo hold of an overnight Air France flight bound for Paris.

The samples then made their way to two labs, one at the Institut Pasteur in Paris, and one in Lyon that could also test for hemorrhagic fever. Formenty called the lab in Lyon to ask them to test the samples for Ebola.[9]

The following morning, Sylvain Baize, an infectious disease expert at the Institut Pasteur, had identified a virus family called filoviruses in the samples, though he could not be certain exactly what species of virus was present. He alerted the World Health Organization, then went back into the lab. By that evening, he had found evidence of Ebola.[10] Hours later, on March 22, 2014, nearly four months after Emile had died, WHO officially declared it had confirmed the presence of Ebola in Guinea. They did not warn of potential cases that had yet to be confirmed in Liberia or Sierra

Leone; it would be months before they confirmed those countries were infected.

The first situational report issued by WHO, three days later, showed just how quickly the virus had spread: it showed eighty-six total cases of Ebola in Guinea and fifty-nine deaths.

By the time the world knew that the flame spreading across the Forest Region was Ebola, eight villages and cities were on fire. And while earlier outbreaks quickly ebbed for lack of new hosts, this epidemic was about to find new fuel. A few days earlier, the same day the Ebola-tainted blood left Conakry for Paris, a trader who made his living exchanging goods in the Forest Region arrived in Conakry.[11] He was not feeling well; he had a fever.

T W O

A Mysterious Killer

MOST VIRUSES, VIEWED UNDER a microscope, have a kind of beauty to them. Some are round, others crystalline, many symmetrical. They inspire an appreciation of the beauty of nature, even if their appearance masks their danger.

The Ebola virus is not beautiful. A member of the filovirus family, it extends in a long, unbroken line, filaments sprouting out like stubbly hairs, wrapping around itself like a coiled snake. It is made of only about 19,000 segments of RNA, the genetic code that governs its existence, a relatively tiny number by comparison to other viruses. A single virion is about 1,000 nanometers in length; it would take about 100 Ebola virions, laid end to end, to match the diameter of a single human hair. Not much is known about Ebola when it is not present in humans, including the identity of its reservoir host.

The Ebola virus, like all viruses, is an accident of evolution. It lives benignly in its reservoir host, with no ill effects, just like the thousands of organisms that inhabit a healthy human. It is not malicious, it does not seek out human life to end. Rather, it seeks an environment in which to repli-cate itself to survive. But there is something in the genetic language of the virus, something in those 19,000 segments of RNA, that orders it to operate differently when it comes into contact with human cells.

The process of a virus jumping from animals to humans is called zoonosis. About 60 percent of all infectious diseases in human history have come from animals—everything from the Bubonic plague, spread by fleas that live on rats, to Lyme disease, spread by tics, and malaria and the Zika virus, harbored in mosquitoes. The moment zoonosis actually takes place is called a spillover.[1]

Once the spillover occurs and the virus enters the human body, a virion seeks out a red blood cell, which it snags with its tiny filaments. The virion is pulled inside its cell, where it begins to reproduce at a breathtaking pace. Within eighteen hours, the number of Ebola virions in an infected cell reaches a critical mass, causing the cell to erupt and shoot thousands of new virions into the bloodstream, where they seek out other cells to infect. They are happiest when they find macrophages, white blood cells that scoop up the remains of dying cells, along with any foreign disease that might have killed them. The Ebola virus, in effect, turns the body's garbage trucks against it—each macrophage another log on the fire, ready to burn, explode—and further spread the invader.

The disease attacks virtually every part of the human body, with the exception of bones and skeletal muscles. It finds particularly attractive cells that line blood vessels in the liver. The infected cells die, dissolving tissues inside the human body.

Ebola is deadly, but compared with other viruses it is relatively difficult to transmit from one human to another. Only when the bodily fluids of an infected person come into contact with a mucus membrane of an uninfected person—whether through the eyeball, the mouth, or an open cut— can the virus jump. Someone who has Ebola but shows no symptoms is not contagious. Even when they are contagious, the disease must travel inside bodily fluids; it is not airborne.

But the virus's ravenous appetite for human tissue means a victim becomes more and more infectious as Ebola finds more and more sustenance. At the moment of death, an infected body is at its most dangerous. Touching the body of an Ebola victim is like stepping on a biological land mine.

In modern history, major outbreaks of hemorrhagic fevers like Ebola have only erupted a handful of times. The first occurred in 1967, when a handful of workers in Marburg, Frankfurt, and Belgrade fell ill after handling infected monkey tissues. Seven of the thirty-one people who fell ill in that first outbreak—a filovirus that came to be known as Marburg—died.

But filoviruses are tens of thousands, maybe millions, of years old. Some historians believe the plague described by the Greek historian Thucydides, which wiped out thousands of Athenians, may have been Ebola. The symptoms Thucydides described match those of Ebola:

> People in good health were all of a sudden attacked by violent heats in the head, and redness and inflammation in the eyes, the inward parts, such as the throat or tongue, becoming bloody and emitting an unnatural and fetid breath. . . . When it fixed in the stomach, it upset it; and discharges of bile of every kind named by physicians ensued, accompanied by very great distress. . . . Internally it burned so that the patient could not bear to have on him clothing or linen even of the very lightest description; or indeed to be otherwise than stark naked.

Thucydides, who contracted and survived the disease himself, said the plague began "in the parts of Ethiopia above Egypt, and thence descended into Egypt and Libya and into most of the King's country."[2]

The first confirmed cases of Ebola in modern history occurred nearly forty years before Emile fell ill, more than 3,000 miles away from West Africa.

In the winter months of 1976, in the small village of Yambuku, in what was then Zaire, Mabalo Lokela fell ill. Lokela was the popular headmaster of Yambuku's only school. When he was taken to the small Catholic mission hospital, run by a team of Belgian nuns who had provided medical treatment to the 60,000 or so residents of the surrounding area since 1935, his fever was spiking. Fluids were leaking from his body faster than medical workers could replace them. He was dead before anyone had time to consider what had killed him.

Then the first wave began. Nearly two dozen patients crowded the hospital, overwhelming doctors who had no idea what they were seeing. The medical staff tried everything in their limited arsenal, from aspirin to chloroquine, nivaquine, stimulants, caffeine, coagulants, anything they could get their hands on. Within a week, fourteen of the first twenty or so infected villagers were dead. They died so fast that the district medical director, making his first report of the outbreak to his superiors in Kinshasa, had to cross out the number of dead. Two more patients had died in the few hours it took him to travel the short distance between Yambuku and his district headquarters, where he could report back to his superiors. Within a month, the hospital had run out of antibiotics. The scene was horrifying; blood was everywhere—in projectile vomit, in explosive diarrhea, oozing from noses and eyes. Doctors, those few who had not fallen ill themselves, sent a message to the capital Kinshasa, begging for help. Lokela's wife, eight months pregnant when her husband first visited the hospital, was one of the few survivors.[3]

By the time an international team of virologists and biologists arrived from the United States, France, Canada, Belgium, and South Africa, along with officials from Zaire's Ministry of Health, a month later, the hospital was closed. Most of the doctors were dead. A medical official from the neighboring province told the Westerners that the disease had already spread through at least forty-four villages within fifty miles of Yambuku in less than a month.

To the scientists who arrived in the new hot zone, led by a pioneering epidemiologist from the Centers for Disease Control and Prevention (CDC), the disease looked familiar. It was related to Marburg, the virus first identified almost a decade before in Europe.

But clearly, this bug was more virulent. By the time the international team arrived in October, when the outbreak was dying down, whatever they were looking at had killed 88 percent of its victims—280 of 318 cases—a mortality rate unheard of since the Black Death of the fourteenth century.

The disease was named for the small river that ran near the village, a tributary of a tributary of the mighty Congo, hardly identified on any but the most detailed maps: the Ebola River.

At almost the same time—in fact, just a few months before the outbreak in Zaire—another hemorrhagic fever had announced itself a few hundred miles away, in the town of Nzara just across Zaire's border with Sudan. (Today, Zaire is the Democratic Republic of the Congo. Nzara has been drawn in to South Sudan, the world's newest nation.) This time, it was workers in a cotton factory who presented the first cases. When the fire burned out, about 53 percent of those infected in the towns of Nzara, Maridi, Tembura, and Juba had died.

Lab tests showed that the two diseases were related, and initially, scientists at the World Health Organization believed the outbreak in Sudan may have sparked the outbreak in Zaire. Eventually, they realized they were looking at two closely related, but distinct, bugs: one would later be named Ebola hemorrhagic fever, abbreviated EBOV by infectious disease researchers; the other would be called Sudan virus, or SUDV, of the same Ebola virus family. (Later, the EBOV disease dropped the "hemorrhagic" from its name; hemorrhages only happened in a small handful of cases.) Subsequent outbreaks would identify two more strains, Bundibugyo virus (BDBV) and Reston virus (RESTV), all closely related but genetically distinct.

Those diseases spread through direct contact with bodily fluids, and evolution has conspired to create conditions for that contact—vomiting, bleeding, and diarrhea all contain deadly amounts of the virus. That puts health-care workers who treat patients at particular risk, though the virus can spread through something as simple as touching one's eye. (Thucydides wrote that physicians in Athens who attempted to treat the sick were among the most vulnerable to the disease.)

After the initial outbreaks in Zaire and Sudan, the virus seemed to disappear, with only the occasional flare-up. A recurrence in Nzara and Maridi, sites of the 1976 outbreak in Sudan, claimed 22 lives three years later. EBOV waited until 1994 to announce its presence once again, this time in Gabon, where 31 of the 52 infected patients died; doctors initially misdiagnosed the disease as yellow fever. The following year, 254 people died—81 percent of those infected—in an outbreak in Kikwit, Zaire. In 1996, 21 of 37 people who fell ill in Mayibout, Gabon, died. Gabon suffered another outbreak in 1997, when 45 of 60 people infected in Booue died.[4]

Those early outbreaks in central Africa provided some clues to researchers investigating this new pathogen, hints that the virus lived somewhere in the jungle. Yambuku is buried deep in the Congolese forest. The first patient to fall ill in Kikwit worked in the forest. In Mayibout, 19 of the 21 who died had handled a chimpanzee found dead in the forest by a band of hunters. (Chimpanzees and apes, so genetically similar to humans, are also highly susceptible to Ebola.) The first victim in Booue was also a hunter from a nearby forest camp where a dead chimpanzee had been found.

After two decades lying dormant, the Ebola virus became a regular, if still rare, crisis for public health officials. Uganda experienced its first outbreak, of the Sudan strain of the virus, in 2000. It arrived in Congo, along the border with Gabon, in 2001, then twice more in 2002 and 2003. Between 2007 and 2009, two outbreaks hit the Democratic Republic of the Congo (renamed in 1997) and another hit Uganda.

The outbreaks caused a terrifying mortality rate. The EBOV strain took the highest tolls, killing between 60 percent and 90 percent of those infected. SUDV caused death in between 40 percent and 60 percent of the infected. BDBV killed fewer than half of its victims, between 25 percent and 47 percent, still a shockingly high number. By comparison, Spanish influenza, which is estimated to have killed around 40 million people from 1918 to 1920 had a mortality rate of just 2.5 percent.[5]

But even with yearly outbreaks, Ebola seemed contained. The towns that suffered were deep in the bush, hours removed from their nearest neighbors over rough terrain or long, winding rivers. The virus killed so fast that only occasionally did anyone infected make it far enough away from the epicenter of an outbreak, called a hot zone, to threaten other populations. Only once did the virus cross into a wholly new country—in 1996, when an infected medical professional who had fought the outbreak at Mayibout got on a plane to South Africa. He survived, but a South African nurse who treated him died.[6]

For the most part, the Ebola virus followed a clear pattern: It would flare up, usually taking root in someone who lived or worked in the forest. Local health workers, unprepared for a disease they usually had no experience with, were primarily at risk, as was the index patient's immediate family. But after a handful of cases, and usually after the arrival of international experts who began establishing a familiar routine of quarantines, the virus would find itself at a dead end, burned out among a small population. There was virtually no risk that Ebola could emerge from the jungles of central Africa to threaten any major population centers.

Still, such a frightening virus was almost certain to catch the imagination of the public. The author Richard Preston helped popularize Ebola in his

1994 book *The Hot Zone,* which described terrifyingly gory scenes of human bodies melting away from a tropical pathogen with no known cure.

In his best seller, Preston included the story of a strain of the Ebola virus that had in fact arrived on American soil a few years before. In 1989, monkeys imported from a facility in the Philippines began dying at a warehouse in Reston, Virginia, just miles from Washington, D.C. Those monkeys were found to have the RESTV strain of the disease, though another genetic quirk appears to have rendered that version of the disease harmless to humans. Three workers at the export facility in Manila had antibodies in their blood; the next year, another monkey die-off showed that the disease was present in four Americans in Virginia and Texas. None of those workers showed any symptoms.

Preston's book inspired the 1995 hit movie *Outbreak*—but his description of the disease borrowed liberally from the imagination, overstating both its dangers and its symptoms. To this day, twenty years later, mentioning Preston's name to a virologist or an epidemiologist elicits a shake of the head, an expletive, or both.

Disease experts had studied Ebola since its very first appearances in 1976. But two disasters seemingly unrelated to tropical diseases—the September 11, 2001, terrorist attacks on New York and Washington and the appearance, just weeks later, of mail laced with anthrax sent to several American newspapers and to members of Congress—gave new urgency to the cause. Suddenly, America faced the prospect of bioterrorism attacks, specific and very contagious pathogens unleashed on the public in confined spaces, like subways or theaters. There was evidence, too, that at least one other nation had pursued research into Ebola, possibly for use in biological weapons: lab workers in Russia had been infected, most likely by accidental needle pricks, in 1996 and 2004. In both cases, those workers died.

Fears of biological threats from abroad spurred the American government to begin studying spreadable diseases with renewed vigor. Working in sealed labs at the Centers for Disease Control and Prevention in Atlanta, the U.S. Army Medical Research Institute for Infectious Diseases (USAMRIID) at Fort Detrick, Maryland, and in a remote National Institutes of Health facility in Hamilton, Montana, scientists studied what they called Category A agents, highly infectious pathogens that could cause widespread outbreaks like smallpox, botulism, tularemia, plague, and hemorrhagic fevers like Marburg, Lassa, and Ebola.

"Our work on Ebola antedated, by many years, the Ebola outbreak, because it was part of something that we started in earnest right after 9/11, when the anthrax attacks occurred in the fall of 2001," said Anthony Fauci, director of the National Institute of Allergy and Infectious Diseases, a division of the National Institutes of Health (NIH). "We put together a program to better understand diseases, at that time based on the perceived need for defense against bioweapons that the Soviet Union had developed during the Cold War."

Much of that work took place at USAMRIID, housed in a patchwork series of stitched-together buildings behind several layers of security at Fort Detrick. Originally designed for just three hundred of the Army's top scientists, it is now home to about a thousand experts and administrators, some crammed into offices that were once called temporary, when they were first installed decades ago.

Below the office space, tucked away off cramped hallways where biohazard suits hang on racks like overcoats for a moon mission, are the laboratories where some of the deadliest diseases in the world are studied. There are four levels of biosafety suites, requiring various protections and protocols depending on how dangerous the substances inside may be. Biosafety level one, or BSL-1, is the equivalent of a classroom, where no special precautions are needed. BSL-2 requires a lab coat, though nothing too hazardous is present.

BSL-3 suites are where the truly dangerous diseases start showing up. Researchers use respirators, masks, and extra gloves to study diseases like Rift Valley Fever, yellow fever, West Nile virus, and severe acute respiratory syndrome (SARS)—diseases that have the potential to be deadly, but for which there are known cures, vaccines, or treatments.

Studying diseases that have no known cures is reserved for specially trained researchers under biosafety level-four conditions, with heavy security and even heavier protections. The BSL-4 suites, visible along white, sterile hallways through double-paned glass, are where Ebola and Marburg live.

Anyone entering one of those suites must pass through three levels of security—a fingerprint scan and two pads that demand unique pin codes— before even entering a changing room. Once there, a researcher will don scrubs before spending several minutes testing a pressurized suit, first visually, and then for any pressure loss. A double submarine door held shut by 6,000 pounds of pressure still stands between the dressing room and the laboratory; neither door can be open when the other is, to ensure a constant barrier between pathogens and the outside world. There are similar precautions inside the laboratory. The room itself has a negative airflow, meaning air is always being sucked in, never pumped directly out. All liquids that leave the laboratory zip through high-pressure lines and come into contact several times with chlorine; both the pressure and the chlorine will kill any potential pathogens left alive. Wastewater is then pumped to a separate holding tank, where it encounters even more chlorine. When lab work is finished, a researcher spends seven minutes in a shower, sprayed down by both water and microchemicals that can kill any living specimen that might remain on the suit.

The suits themselves are cumbersome; the air pumped in from tubes attached to a lab ceiling is loud, and it fills the suit like a balloon, making simple tasks ungainly. Researchers wear earplugs to protect themselves from the noise. Before being allowed to operate in a level-four atmosphere, students train in an unused BSL-4 lab classroom called the Slammer, where they practice building with children's blocks, or rearranging a deck of playing cards. One room of the Slammer even has the game Operation, which helps test dexterity. The students will eventually operate in laboratories where rats and primates are infected with the planet's deadliest diseases. One scientist dropped a casual hint about monkeys fighting off the Ebola virus in some back room. The author was not allowed into that back room.

The research conducted at USAMRIID, CDC, and NIH produced results: A decade after the anthrax attacks, NIH scientists had created a possible vaccine, and early trials were conducted among volunteers from the Washington area, and in close American allies in Africa like Mali, Kenya, and Uganda.

It also produced an intriguing scientific mystery. Scientists from USAMRIID, the Army's chief medical laboratory, had been studying hemorrhagic fever in West Africa for years, led by Dr. Randy Schoepp, aided by a team from Tulane University, headed by Dr. Robert Garry, and a private pharmaceutical company based in San Francisco called Metabiota.

They set up shop at a hospital in Kenema, Sierra Leone's third-largest city, where they built the world's only ward dedicated to treating Lassa.

Kenema, near the border with Liberia, had long played an important role in scientists' struggle to understand viral hemorrhagic fevers, specifically Lassa. The CDC had set up an outpost at Kenema Government Hospital in the 1970s, where some of the earliest work on the rodent-borne disease took place. (The first CDC investigator to be deployed to Kenema, Joe McCormick, hadn't even gotten a chance to unpack his equipment from its shipping containers before he was temporarily diverted to Yambuku, to fight the Ebola outbreak there.[7])

But many of the samples of possible Lassa cases Schoepp and Garry were seeing were testing negative. Of the five hundred to seven hundred suspected Lassa cases in Sierra Leone in the years between 2006 and 2008, which Schoepp analyzed, only about 30 to 40 percent were testing positive. The rest of the victims had suffered from something else—some other hemorrhagic disease that was present, albeit on the margins, in the jungles of West Africa. Schoepp's team isolated the antibodies, a body's response to the presence of a pathogen: They looked remarkably similar to Ebola antibodies. Garry's research indicated that similar antibodies had been present in the region for up to a decade.

That did not make sense. Unlike Uganda, Gabon, Congo, and the Democratic Republic of the Congo in Central Africa, West Africa had only ever seen one confirmed case of Ebola, when a Swiss graduate student working on dead chimpanzees in a national park in Côte d'Ivoire fell ill. The student had contracted a new strain of the disease, called the Tai Forest strain, or TAFV; she survived. The TAFV strain has never been documented in another human.

Schoepp's team initially believed they had found new evidence of the TAFV strain of the virus. But the more they studied the antibodies, the more they concluded they might be looking at the much more deadly EBOV strain. "That was a good indication to us that there was Ebola Zaire circulating in Sierra Leone, Guinea, and Liberia" before the 2014 outbreak, Schoepp said later.

Few believed him, and the rigors of scientific research precluded Schoepp from reaching a definitive conclusion. Though the antibodies were present, scientists could not isolate a strain of the virus itself, meaning they could not prove without a doubt that Ebola Zaire was present. "Nobody believed there was Ebola in West Africa," Schoepp said. Still, he concluded, it was likely that Ebola had broken out, possibly routinely but never disastrously, long before 2014. Garry believed he had evidence that showed Ebola had started small, infecting just a few people a year, then grown and grown. The question in his mind was not whether one of those minor outbreaks would spread and kill thousands—but when.

By the time the NIH's vaccine was in phase one tests, gauging the safety and effectiveness, called immunogenicity, in humans, Emile was sick. And unlike earlier outbreaks, Ebola began speeding toward major population centers.

That Ebola would migrate thousands of miles away to those three countries seemed at first to be an almost impossible stroke of bad luck. The colonial powers that departed from West Africa in the 1950s and 1960s left behind two countries—Sierra Leone, once a part of the British Empire, and Guinea, a French colony—in desperately poor shape. Both powers had treated their African subjects terribly; French colonizers forced Guineans to build roads and tap rubber trees, and the British used Sierra Leone and what is now Liberia as the base of operations for the slave trade from the sixteenth to the nineteenth centuries.

Liberia's own history is even more complex. Established in the nineteenth century as a new home for freed African, African American, and Caribbean slaves, it was the first nation in Africa to formally gain independence, when the United States recognized it in 1862. The freed slaves who returned to Liberia in the nineteenth century did not arrive in an empty land, and occasional battles between indigenous tribes, which make up about 80 percent of the country's population, and the descendants of former slaves cost hundreds of thousands of lives. Even today, Liberia has two parallel governing structures: a formal government, populated largely by descendants of former slaves centered in Monrovia, and a tribal power structure, consisting of a complex hierarchy of town and provincial chiefs, all the way up to a national level. Lower-level officials on the two sides work closely together; the higher up the ranks, the worse the professional relationship.

Formed from the ashes of the Western slave trade, struggling to recover from decades of internal strife and tribal conflict, the three nations are impoverished even by African standards. They are tied together by history, thanks to Western meddling and centuries of tribal ties, and by geography. On a map, Guinea seems to enfold the other two nations, the artificial borders drawn by European hands, the results of an agreement formalized in 1895, thousands of miles away at a signing ceremony attended by colonial British and French diplomats in Paris. Guinea's capital, Conakry, is the northernmost of the three; Guinea wraps east into the interior, then around its two neighbors. Sierra Leone lies south of Guinea, its own southern border shared with Liberia. All three capitals, Conakry, Freetown, and Monrovia, founded by Europeans and Americans centuries ago, face the Atlantic Ocean.

Death is no stranger to West Africa. All three countries have been torn apart by civil wars and ruthless dictators. All three have supported insurgencies in their neighbors. Up to half a million Liberians died in civil wars between 1989 and 1997, then again between 2000 and 2003, in which rebels funded by Sierra Leone and Guinea clashed with the government run by the brutal Charles Taylor. About 50,000 Sierra Leoneans died in a decade-long civil war that ended in 2001; United Nations peacekeeping troops spent the following five years disarming rebel groups, before leaving in 2005. Guinea's president Ahmed Sekou Toure funded wars across the region.

On a continent with a long and deadly history of colonial rule, the three West African nations are unique, both for their dependence and independence. Portuguese traders first explored the coast of West Africa in the late fifteenth century. The explorer Pedro da Cintra was the first to name the mountains near the coast, which he called the Lion Mountains, or Serra Lyoa in his native tongue. Other colonizers would eventually exert their own spheres of influence. The first British settlements were established in Sierra Leone in the mid-1600s, from which raiders kidnapped Africans to send to the new world. The first African slaves arrived in North America in the middle of the seventeenth century. French troops established themselves in what is now Guinea about a century and a half later, marauding through the interior attacking the Malinke tribe.

Early movements to find new homes for freed black slaves in Britain and the United States gave birth to modern Sierra Leone and Liberia. In

1792, the Committee for the Relief of the Black Poor sent 1,200 free blacks on 15 ships from British-controlled Nova Scotia to establish a colony christened Free Town. In 1822, the first ship carrying 37 settlers and 10 liberated slaves from the Virginia colony arrived on Cape Montserado, which had been purchased from a local tribal chief by the American Colonization Society. Within the next decade, another 2,600 freed blacks moved from America to the new town, first called Christopolis, then renamed Monrovia—the only capital of a foreign country to be named after an American president, James Monroe, who helped secure a $100,000 congressional appropriation to establish the settlement. (The movement to send freed blacks back to Africa represented a duality of purpose in both Britain and the United States. On one hand, there was a growing population of abolitionists committed to ending slavery and freeing African slaves. On the other, those same abolitionists preferred that the newly freed blacks leave America or Britain, rather than staying and living among their white neighbors.)

The American Colonization Society struggled to pay the bills for the new colonies they established around Monrovia. By 1847, they urged the colonies, since joined together, to declare themselves the independent nation of Liberia. Though the United States continued to keep a close eye on the tiny country, Liberia was the only nation in Africa not to be colonized by a European power.

Still, the so-called repatriation of freed African slaves was nothing of the sort. Those who left America to return to Africa were culturally, ethnically, and linguistically distinct from the tribesmen who had called Liberia their home for millennia. After establishing the new nation, the colonists, repressed for generations themselves, denied the indigenous population the right to vote unless they converted to Christianity. After a century of rampant embezzlement of foreign funds, three decades of violence began in 1980 with the violent overthrow of President William Tolbert. Civil war raged, pitting tribes against the class of descendants of American slaves, and tribes against tribes; almost every effort at peace failed until 2005, when a former World Bank economist named Ellen Johnson Sirleaf won election, promising national reconciliation.

Sierra Leone declared its independence from the United Kingdom in 1961. Guinea emerged from the ashes of France's Fourth Republic in 1958, when new prime minister Charles de Gaulle made clear to French colonies they could declare independence. Both nations struggled: Sierra Leone's government was toppled three times in a period of two years in the late 1960s. The one-party rule of President Toure sent 200,000 Guineans fleeing into exile. After Toure's death in 1984, a military coup landed another strongman, Lansana Conte, in power until his death in 2008. His elected successor, Alpha Conde—a former opposition leader who fled into exile after Lansana Conte jailed him for eight months in 2001—has delayed parliamentary elections since taking office in 2010.

Even though other African nations suffered under colonial rule, the decades—centuries—of violence in the three West African nations left their populations among the poorest in the world. Dry statistics only hint at the poverty that strangles West Africa. In 2013, Guinea's per capita gross domestic product (GDP) was only $521; Sierra Leone's was $797; and Liberia's was just $453. The same year, the per capita GDP of the United States was $52,980, according to the World Bank.[8] Just over 30 percent of Guineans and 35 percent of Sierra Leoneans are literate, among the lowest rates in the world. The life expectancy in Sierra Leone, forty-six years, is ranked 194th on a list of 194 countries studied by the World Bank; Guineans can expect to live fifty-eight years on average, 172nd on the list. Liberians live to be sixty-two, on average, seventeen years less than the average American. Just 1 percent of the population of all three countries has access to the Internet.

To the ethnic groups that dominate the three West African nations, the new borders, artificially drawn based on European whims, meant little—other than that rivals with centuries of antagonistic history were thrown together in one country, and that allied tribes with deep familial ties were divided by some faceless French or British cartographer. Civil wars erupted once colonizers left. And even today, remote tribes living at the intersection of all three countries ignore border lines on irrelevant maps, crossing freely to do business and see family in neighboring towns.

After centuries of colonization and decades of war, Liberia, Sierra Leone, and Guinea were left destitute. Few nongovernmental organizations were present. American aid continued to flow to Liberia, in particular, through the United States Agency for International Development, but extreme poverty had decimated the national health-care systems in all three countries. Those health systems were so underfunded and ill-prepared that even basic medical care was impossible: Public health experts estimate a nation needs to have 22.8 medical professionals—doctors, nurses, midwives, and others—for every 10,000 residents, just to provide basic levels of care. Before the outbreak, Sierra Leone had just five professionals for every 10,000 residents.

It was into this atmosphere, this tinderbox, that the spark of Ebola landed. Suddenly, the nations that the international community had ignored for so long demanded immediate attention.

THREE

Into the Fight

FOR DAYS IN THE middle of March 2014, the global health community held its breath, waiting for confirmation from the French laboratories that the fire raging through the Forest Region was Ebola. The virus didn't bother to wait; it spread, first across the border to Liberia, then closer and closer to the largest cities in West Africa.

Tewa Joseph, who had carried her sister Tamba to the hospital in Foya-Borma, fell ill the same day Tamba died. By the time she arrived at the same hospital, doctors and nurses knew a killer disease was in their midst— and they had no protection from its spread. They refused the young woman admission. New cases began appearing faster than Guinea's already-insufficient health system could cope: by March 27, 103 cases had been reported. By the thirty-first, 9 new cases were confirmed. On April 1, 10 more patients were identified, the next day, 5 more, and 25 more in the following 5 days, in Guinea alone.

The mortality rate shocked local officials. By April 7, of the 151 cases reported in Guinea, 95 people had died.

But while an Ebola outbreak was unprecedented in West Africa, the global community's response was well-practiced. And once the World Health Organization (WHO) announced the presence of Ebola in Guinea, virus hunters reprised their familiar roles. After two dozen or so outbreaks across central Africa, the early moves were so familiar they happened as muscle memory. Epidemiologists and virologists from Africa, Europe, and the United States rounded up their equipment, jumped on planes, and descended on the hot zone. Those with years of practice quarantining and treating patients and hunting for the Ebola virus in nearby forests began arriving in Conakry, Guinea's capital. Many, seeing old friends and occasional rivals at the relatively posh Palm Camayenne Hotel, exchanged hugs.[1]

In the United States, the Centers for Disease Control and Prevention (CDC) dispatched its first team, including some of the most experienced Ebola responders in the world. President Obama heard about the outbreak for the first time on March 24, when officials from the Central Intelligence Agency included a mention of the WHO's declaration in his morning security briefing. The first American tasked with marshaling a response to the epidemic would be Michael Schmoyer, director of the Office of Security and Strategic Information, a division of the Department of Health and Human Services.

Médecins Sans Frontières, or MSF, already had a presence in Guinea, where they had been vaccinating residents against cholera and malaria. Just a day after WHO declared Ebola present, an MSF team opened its first Ebola treatment facility in Gueckedou, near the virus's epicenter. Two days later, MSF opened its first Ebola Management Center, a higher-tech facility, at Donka Hospital in Conakry; over the next year, that facility would admit and treat more than 1,800 patients.

The same day, Dr. Stephane Hugonnet, a senior WHO official in charge of global capacities, alert and responses, landed in Guinea to oversee the response. WHO brought a mobile lab to Gueckedou, capable of testing up to fifty blood samples a day.[2]

In neighboring Liberia, another nongovernmental organization (NGO), Global Communities, worried about the possible spread across an international border. Piet deVries and Brett Sedgewick, two veterans of decades of disaster relief operations in some of Africa's most war-torn environments, led the group's operations in Liberia, where it ran a water sanitation program in remote rural counties hours by car from Monrovia. DeVries called his counterparts at WHO to offer help, and within days, Global Communities trucks were racing supplies north to Lofa County, just across from the affected region.

In a culture where the very concept of viral disease is virtually unknown, many of those rural residents believed Ebola was little more than a ruse. Rumors in Gueckedou and the surrounding communities mounted almost the moment the first Ebola treatment facilities were opened. Some watched their relatives enter the mysterious white tents, manned by foreigners in what looked like space suits. Those relatives never came out. When those who nursed their loved ones fell ill themselves, some refused to go to a treatment center. Others tried to escape from medical facilities, carrying the disease with them.

In a way, the international community's response to an Ebola outbreak was so well-practiced that it caused problems. The men and women in space suits showed up before news of the outbreak reached local communities. The fraught relationship between the government in Monrovia and the rural communities run by tribal elders made some question whether this wasn't an elaborate plot—or worse. Was this disease real, some villagers wondered, or had these Westerners in space suits brought it with them? Virus-hunting teams sent to some small settlements were chased away by angry crowds.

In Liberia, the historical disconnect between the tribesmen who inhabited remote rural counties and the descendants of former slaves who ran the government in Monrovia picked apart a scab that never fully healed after the deadly civil war a decade earlier. But that distrust between governments and tribes was not unique to Liberia. Guinea's president, Alpha Conde, was a member of the Malinke ethnic group, which made up about 15 percent of the nation's 10 million residents. The majority Fula ethnic group were suspicious that Conde was using the virus as cover to delay an upcoming election (indeed, the election was delayed). Some in the Kissi tribe, an impoverished and persecuted minority who inhabited the Forest Region that straddled all three countries, believed the virus had been introduced to exterminate them.[3]

Some villages would not admit Ebola was in their midst at all. The poor health systems in Guinea and Liberia had weak, or nonexistent, diagnostic capabilities, so who could say what had killed someone? "In Liberia," deVries explained, "there's a lot of unknown death."

Government officials in all three countries were terrified, too, that the presence of the disease could deliver another devastating blow to their economies. International corporations had only recently begun investing in Guinea, Liberia, and Sierra Leone; the last thing any of those countries and their beleaguered economies needed was evidence of new unrest.

That threat inspired denial at the highest levels of government. Four days after the first confirmed case in Guinea, and the day Liberia's second Ebola case, Tewa Joseph, was being refused entry to the hospital in Foya-Borma, the Liberian Information, Culture and Tourism minister Lewis Brown told a local newspaper that his country was virus-free.[4] The next day, WHO reported eight cases in Liberia, six of whom had died.

The Liberian Ministry of Health, which had held a press conference on March 24 to report on suspected cases, suddenly stopped referring to Ebola at all. The Forest Region, ministry officials said, only showed signs of a "suspected viral hemorrhagic fever."[5] Dr. Aboubacar Sidiki Diakite, the Guinean health official in charge of beating back the outbreak, insisted on counting only those who had tested positive for Ebola among the country's roster of total cases, rather than including all suspected cases, even though testing facilities were working painfully slowly and some patients were obviously infected.

The WHO itself received strong pressure from West African governments. In one early conference call with global health responders, including several top American medical officials, a senior WHO official downplayed the threat. "We don't want to make this out to be a real big problem," the official said. "It'll be a terrible problem for tourism and stigma."

Anthony Fauci, participating in the call from his office at the National Institute of Allergy and Infectious Diseases at the National Institutes of Health outside Washington, almost fell off his chair, so shocked that tourism was a concern in the face of one of the world's most deadly diseases.

"There was a certain amount of reluctance to accept the severity of the problem," WHO's Chris Dye recalled later, employing British understatement to the fullest degree. Margaret Chan, WHO's director general, was on the phone with all three heads of state on a weekly basis, urging aggressive action. Her calls with Fauci, CDC director Tom Frieden, and others in the United States were becoming more frequent, too.

Even the most determined efforts to deny the virus's presence fell short, and the world took note. On April 1, Saudi Arabia announced it would stop issuing visas for Guinean and Liberian Muslims who wanted to participate in an *umrah* or a hajj, the traditional pilgrimages to Mecca, Islam's holiest city. Three days later, an Air France flight from Conakry was quarantined on the runway at Charles de Gaulle Airport in Paris after a passenger threw up in an onboard lavatory. Every passenger was checked for fever as they disembarked.[6]

Not everyone worried about the financial bottom line. On March 27, five days after the virus was formally identified, Peter Sonpon Coleman, chairman of the Liberian Senate's committee responsible for health, made the first request for money to fight an outbreak that was almost certain to cross into his country. He asked for $1.2 million.[7]

Outside of government structures, the virus was spreading. The trader who had arrived in Conakry with a fever had infected others, including some of the precious few health-care workers trying desperately to prop up Guinea's terribly poor health system. When Rob Fowler, the Canadian physician dispatched by the WHO, arrived at Kipe Hospital in Conakry, he found that most of the likely Ebola patients were health-care workers. Just one nurse and a handful of doctors had managed to escape infection. None had been trained to take the precautions necessary when treating a suspected or confirmed Ebola patient. His reaction, he wrote later, was "no small amount of fear."[8] Across the entire city, a metropolis of 1.6 million, just four doctors and four nurses were treating Ebola patients.

By the beginning of April, MSF had established themselves as the NGO with the greatest capacity to mount the initial medical response. The group opened new Ebola isolation wards in Macenta and Conakry; sixty workers were dispatched, along with forty tons of equipment.[9] But even those doctors, well-known in Guinea, were subject to local skeptics, some of whom turned violent. An Ebola surveillance team was chased out of one neighborhood in Macenta by an angry crowd; the crowd then smashed in the brand-new treatment center, too.

Hugonnet, the WHO official, was among the first to realize the extent of the public relations campaign the international organizations needed to mount. Ebola, after all, was unknown in West Africa, so much so that even the medical experts who had visited Meliandou several months earlier had not recognized what they were looking at. Now, as the disease spread, international organizations were going to have to find a way to communicate a few specific themes: The disease was real. It was deadly. But it was treatable.

It fell to Cristiana Salvi, a WHO communications specialist, to begin crafting that message in hard-hit Gueckedou. Salvi's arrival in the city, population about 79,000, in late April, underscored its remoteness. Her tiny plane bounced along a rutted runway, seemingly in the middle of nowhere, that served as the regional airport. From there, a car lurched over even worse roads for two hours before Gueckedou emerged from the forest.[10]

Salvi was concerned that the messages Guinean authorities were spreading were not sufficiently tailored to those most likely to come into contact with Ebola. Those messages were largely the same as the ones spread in the Democratic Republic of the Congo and other countries that had been hit by the disease before. Residents in hot zones were told to give up some common practices that brought them into close contact with the disease, like washing bodies before burial. That worked in the Congo, where Ebola was known. In Guinea, no one knew what it was that killed their relatives. To distrusting villagers, the initial message sounded like Westerners interfering with centuries of cultural tradition.

The lack of knowledge about and experience with Ebola meant a basic education campaign was crucial. Women were especially at risk because cultural expectations in Guinea and Liberia held that women care for the sick, and then prepare the dead for burial. That meant women were coming into direct contact with Ebola victims at their most contagious stage.

Salvi and her colleagues began crafting a message, informed by focus groups, that would introduce Ebola as a danger, one with a massively high fatality rate. Radio advertising and billboards were soon ubiquitous around Gueckedou and other parts of Guinea.

Some of the new procedures and protocols took hold. When Piet deVries met with a county health official in Lofa County, just across the border from Guinea, in late March, he put out his hand, ready for the customary Liberian handshake, half high-five, with a snap at the end. The health official just looked at him: handshaking was already forbidden.

But the initial message, Salvi later wrote, worked at counter purposes to the WHO's goals. Warning of Ebola's extreme danger gave Guineans the impression they would not survive if they were infected—and dying at home surrounded by family would be infinitely better than dying in a hot, fetid, putrid hospital surrounded by Westerners in moon suits. "Most of the people who catch [Ebola] will die," read one poster. Other messages missed the point completely: Liberian and Guinean health ministry advertising urged villagers to avoid eating bush meat, or plums that had been nibbled by bats; epidemiologically, villagers did not have to worry about catching Ebola from the wild, they had to worry about catching it from their friends and relatives. Once again, patients began disappearing before they could be taken to an Ebola treatment center. Groups like Samaritan's Purse, one of the first outside NGOs to arrive in the hot zone, pleaded with health ministries to change their messages.

So Salvi crafted a new message, one that highlighted survivors. Though they were few, at the outbreak's initial phase, there were some. They proved Ebola was not necessarily a death sentence if a victim sought treatment early enough. In advertisements and in newspaper stories, survivors shared their experiences—how they were infected, how they were treated, and, just as important, how they were fed as they recovered. Communicators on WHO's staff had to convince the communities they were trying to reach the basic fact that they were there to help, not to spread the mysterious disease within the community.

The groups fighting Ebola on the ground in Gueckedou, and increasingly in Conakry, needed to communicate beyond those who were infected. They needed to reach those patients' families, who had to deliver them to hospitals. Early on, families were given disposable cell phones so they could contact their loved ones inside an isolation unit. Families were also given money for taxis to visit their relatives in person, even if they were separated by the plastic walls of a treatment center.

The race to set up clinics was a logistical nightmare. The few medical professionals who lived and worked in the rural settings where Ebola now raged knew nothing of diseases that could be so easily transmitted between humans. They were accustomed to other deadly pathogens—cholera, malaria—that were ubiquitous, but not contagious.

That meant the frontline clinics, where Ebola patients would first encounter the medical system, needed upgrades, and fast. The supplies Piet deVries and his team at Global Communities raced north included only the most basic personal protection equipment—PPEs, in epidemiological shorthand. They brought thousands of body bags, gallons of chlorine to disinfect any surface on which Ebola might survive, and crates filled with gloves and masks.

The need for even basic supplies was acute. In some more remote areas, gloves, life-saving essentials for any medical professional, began selling for the equivalent of fifty cents a pair, in an area where most residents lived on less than a dollar a day.

Nongovernmental organizations worked hard, too, to convince villagers that Ebola was real, not some curse cast by rivals, not some trick of a sinister government. Global Communities was the only NGO to have operated for such a long period of time in rural counties, meaning that their employees had credibility with villagers and, more important, with tribal leaders. Their decade-long campaign to change sanitation behavior by demonstrating a link between open defecation near water sources and cholera—a program called Community-Led Total Sanitation, or CLTS—had been implemented by hundreds of environmental health technicians.

Now, those technicians, so used to demonstrating how to dig a safe latrine, were pressed into far more dangerous circumstances. Through April, May, and June, the technicians held dozens of meetings at clinics around Lofa, Bong, and Nimba Counties, where they helped village leaders develop action plans and response activities.

At the same time, the United States Agency for International Development (USAID) and its partners at UNICEF began their own massive education campaign, and their own networks of tribal leaders. USAID and UNICEF helped tribal chiefs, women's groups, and others spread the word about Ebola in their own villages.

However late it was, the international response, five months after Emile came down with a terrible fever, had finally come to the rescue. By mid-May, the familiar pattern of an Ebola outbreak appeared to show itself: daily case counts began to slow, and some previously suspected cases turned out to be something else. The total number of cases in Guinea continued to grow, but at a slower pace. Over the last week of April and the first week of May, just ten new cases were reported. By April 9 Liberia isolated the last of the dozen cases that initially broke out on their side of the border. A few weeks later, the country went three weeks with only one new case. Sierra Leone, which experienced one scare in late March, had not reported a single new case.

Still, as the global health community descended on Guinea and Liberia, the power of a virus so small weighed on those first responders. By the end of April, a month after WHO confirmed that Ebola had begun to kill, 234 people had been infected. Of those, 157 had died.

FOUR

A Turning Point

EVERY VIRUS, LIKE A fire, can only survive as long as it has a fuel source. The speed with which a virus consumes its fuel source determines just how long the outbreak's lifespan extends. What scared epidemiologists during that chaotic first month, when the Ebola outbreak migrated from Meliandou to Gueckedou and then toward more densely populated urban areas in both Guinea and Liberia, was that the virus had apparently found a fuel source far greater than ever before. Conakry and Monrovia are large, terribly impoverished cities, where hundreds of thousands of residents live in densely packed slums. These were not the remote jungles of the Congo, where previous outbreaks had erupted and then calmed for lack of anyone else to infect; they were perfect fuel sources for a voracious virus in search of new human hosts.

But in the chaos of those early days, the global health community's initial response to the Ebola outbreak was muted and confused, even as the virus worked toward urban centers.

On the surface, the race to contain one of the world's deadliest diseases appeared robust: World Health Organization (WHO) foot soldiers from Geneva and around the globe arrived within days. Médecins Sans Frontières (MSF), or Doctors Without Borders, shipped tons of supplies and hundreds of their own volunteers. The first Americans, including some of the world's most qualified Ebola responders dispatched by the Centers for Disease Control and Prevention (CDC) in Atlanta, parachuted in just days later.

But the rapid activity masked a deep, disturbing reality: The global health network was completely unprepared to respond to an outbreak of the magnitude now spreading from rural villages toward West Africa's largest cities. And even though the outbreak threatened to become the largest, most widespread emergence of Ebola in world history, its seriousness did nothing to stop the squabbling—some of it alarmingly sophomoric—among the response groups that arrived in late March and early April of 2014.

The internal fights began almost the moment scientists confirmed Ebola's presence. On March 31, just a week after confirmation, senior MSF officials realized what they faced. Already, the international organization had sixty staffers on the ground, including doctors, nurses, epidemiologists, and sanitation experts, and the data they were collecting was terrifying. New cases had sprouted up all over, from remote Gueckedou to urban Conakry.

"We are facing an epidemic of a magnitude never before seen in terms of the distribution of cases in the country," warned Mariano Lugli, MSF's coordinator in Conakry. The group's headquarters staff, in a press release, called the outbreak "unprecedented." A Twitter message warned that the strain of Ebola detected in Guinea, EBOV, had a mortality rate of up to 90 percent.

In Geneva, WHO officials bristled at what they saw as MSF's alarmism. "Don't exaggerate," WHO spokesman Gregory Hartl tweeted in response to MSF's warning of the extremely high mortality rate.[1] In another Twitter message, Hartl downplayed the seriousness of the early spread: "You want to disrupt the economic life of a country, a region [because] of 130 suspect and confirmed cases?" he sneered.

MSF officials were aghast. Here was the top spokesman for the World Health Organization, the international body ostensibly in charge of fighting back against these outbreaks, seemingly playing games with one of the most deadly viruses on the planet.

Those who counted on WHO to organize a robust response quickly became disillusioned. The organization, based in Geneva, is not built to orchestrate a global response to a massive crisis—or even a small crisis—and it has neither the authority nor the funding to do so. For years, Margaret Chan and others had been begging donor countries to fully fund WHO's budget for just such an occasion as a massive outbreak of a deadly virus. For years, donor countries, including the United States, had cut their commitments instead. What's more, WHO simply isn't built as a worldwide response operation.

"We're a really normative agency. We gather scientific evidence and provide advice on the nature of ill health," Chris Dye, WHO's director for Strategy, Policy and Information, said later. "We're not typically an operational agency. In other words, we don't do what the World Food Programme does. We don't do what UNICEF does. We're not in the trenches."

Pierre Formenty, one of the world's top Ebola experts, experienced WHO's lack of standing and authority firsthand. He was part of WHO's initial team of thirty-eight dispatched to fight the outbreak in Guinea. When he landed in Conakry, he was passed over for a role as a team coordinator.[2] The job went, instead, to someone who had never been involved in an Ebola outbreak.

In Atlanta, Tom Frieden watched with growing irritation as petty squabbles overseas delayed his own teams. Several teams were delayed by bureaucratic hurdles, seemingly erected by local WHO officials who wanted to prove they could handle the outbreak themselves. When Pierre Rollin, the CDC's preeminent Ebola expert, arrived in Guinea on April 1, he and four colleagues were delayed in deploying to the field. They spent several days cooped up in their hotel rooms, debugging software that would eventually help responders track the virus to trace those who might have been exposed. Fending off cabin fever, they worked virtually around the clock, toting their computers to dinner in the hotel restaurant, typing as they ate.[3] Rollin busied himself briefing staff at the American, British, and French embassies on the basics of Ebola; a native French speaker, he held a special French language briefing for Guinean drivers and staff, who were most likely to come into contact with the virus when they went home at night.[4]

The delays, the infighting, were a feature, not a bug, in the global health response system—more specifically, in WHO itself.

The World Health Organization was established in 1946 under the auspices of the United Nations to control the spread of deadly diseases like tuberculosis and malaria and to improve health conditions, especially for women and children. The organization was meant to standardize procedures for disease reporting, a crucial factor in finding and eradicating outbreaks. Its main tool was shame: only the WHO could publicize outbreaks of some diseases, under the theory that any country with an outbreak would be forced to respond aggressively or risk lost tourism dollars and economic activity. In many cases, shame worked: the WHO helped eliminate smallpox, and over its seventy years of existence, it has saved countless lives by fighting the spread of measles, HIV/AIDS, and polio, among other deadly scourges.

But WHO is, at its heart, a patron of its client states. While it is headquartered in Geneva, WHO has divided the world into six regions, one on each populated continent. Directors of those regions are appointed by consensus among health ministers on each continent, and the director then appoints a senior WHO official in each of the countries under his or her jurisdiction. That means regional directors are answerable to health ministers, and governments, in their own region—not to the populations served by those governments.

In West Africa, that meant tiptoeing around health and information ministers, the former struggling to deal with a mounting medical crisis, the latter determined to avoid the negative publicity that could drive away millions of dollars in desperately needed economic development and tourism.

"WHO didn't sound the global alarm early or effectively, long after there was plenty of data to demonstrate that [Ebola] was a problem," said Rajiv Shah, then the head of the United States Agency for International Development (USAID). "They were enmeshed in the politics of not wanting to upset a country or a region."

The African region of WHO is headquartered in Brazzaville, in the Republic of the Congo, close enough to the historic range of previous Ebola outbreaks but thousands of miles from West Africa. And the agency, which depends on private donations for about three-quarters of its annual budget, faced the pressures of the global recession just like any other charity: donations dried up, demanding painful budget cuts. In Africa, those budget cuts hit preparedness efforts. Between fiscal year 2010 and fiscal year 2014, the

WHO's epidemic preparedness and response budget plunged, from $26 million annually to just $11 million. Nine of the twelve emergency response specialists the WHO employed in Brazzaville were laid off.[5]

Though some government ministers in Guinea and Liberia downplayed the seriousness of the outbreak, its severity soon required robust responses. The woefully inadequate health care systems left over in West Africa after generations of war just were not capable of delivering those responses. WHO's usual tactic, shame, wouldn't work: Alpha Conde, Guinea's president, and Ellen Johnson Sirleaf, president of Liberia, did the opposite of obscuring the presence of Ebola in their region—they publicly begged for help. Conde traveled to Geneva in late April for consultations with WHO. Johnson Sirleaf was in constant contact with American officials, asking for more aid.

WHO, however, was in no position to provide anything resembling an overwhelming response. Not only had their budget been hammered by the recession, but WHO proved early on it had done little to lay the groundwork necessary to send help when it was needed. There was no list of thousands of volunteer doctors who could help, no list of drugs in early stages of development that could be rushed through the testing and trial process, and no ready supply of materials necessary for building hospitals or mobile labs.

The world had assumed its chief global health watchdog had the capacity to respond to a deadly outbreak. The world had assumed wrong.

No organization worked more aggressively to pick up WHO's slack than MSF.

Where WHO is an internationally sanctioned body, MSF is fiercely independent. It was founded in 1971, after French doctors volunteering with the Red Cross accused the agency of turning a blind eye to the Nigerian army's murder of civilians. Today, MSF is funded almost entirely by private donors; the group will not accept grants from governments like the United States, for fear that taking the money would give the impression that MSF endorsed or condoned a donor government's actions. It operates in the worst conflict zones around the world, from Bosnia and Rwanda in the 1990s to Iraq and Afghanistan today, where its doctors and nurses treat combatants from all sides; in Afghanistan, its hospitals cared for Taliban fighters and government troops, sometimes side by side (MSF had a history in West Africa, too, having responded to the Liberian civil war in 1990).

For a private nonprofit with a limited budget and penny-pinching ways, MSF's actions in West Africa were nothing short of herculean. In the course of a year that the group spent responding to the Ebola outbreak in West Africa, it raised and spent $100 million, dispatched a total of 5,000 staffers, and built and maintained 15 Ebola treatment centers. All told, MSF cared for one in every three people infected with the virus.

At times, however, MSF's altruism grated on the nerves of other responders. When American agencies began introducing some of the drugs it was testing, both possible treatments for those infected with the virus and vaccines designed to protect health care workers from getting infected, MSF officials bristled at the caution with which drug testing took place. If one patient was going to get an experimental drug, MSF believed, all patients should get that drug.

That startled the American agencies that already thought they were moving as fast as was medically responsible in testing potential cures and diagnostic assays.

Those American agencies had been quietly at work on Ebola for more than a decade, since the attacks of September 11, 2001, and subsequent anthrax attacks raised the prospects of a terrorist attack using biological weapons long before the virus arrived in Guinea, Sierra Leone, and Liberia. Both the National Institutes of Health (NIH) and the U.S. Army Medical Research Institute for Infectious Diseases (USAMRIID) had spent more than a decade preparing to respond to an epidemic, whether naturally spread or spread by terrorists.

In 2009, David Norwood, chief of USAMRIID's diagnostics systems division, sat down with top officials at the Food and Drug Administration (FDA), the agency that must approve both drugs and the chemical compounds that would demonstrate proof of a virus's presence.

Those chemical compounds, called assays, work by bonding with a virus's RNA strand, which produces a burst of fluorescent light. The delicate and expensive computers analyzing a sample of blood detect those emissions, which show that the virus is present. Winning approval for a specific assay was easier than getting a new drug approved, but it still required lab results that showed it would work. The problem was that the companies creating the assays could not always show that their compounds worked with diseases like Ebola, because they didn't have any Ebola to test. Only government agencies like the CDC or USAMRIID had samples of the virus, locked away in highly secure biocontainment suites. They were not in the habit of handing out samples of something as deadly as Ebola.

Still, in the event of an outbreak, Norwood told FDA regulators, they would need to move fast. To prepare for whatever came next, Army doctors sent more than seventy assays to the FDA, testing for everything from Ebola and Marburg to anthrax and botulism. The moment a new outbreak cropped up, the appropriate assays would be given immediate priority. Together, the two agencies prepared for an Emergency Use Authorization, a declaration by the secretary of Health and Human Services that would allow them to speed the approval process by skipping a few more rigorous steps, all in hopes of getting the diagnostics to the front lines as fast as possible.

The NIH and CDC had been busy with their own preparations. They had a promising drug to treat Ebola patients, known as Favipiravir, that had already undergone early testing regimens on volunteers in the United States and some African countries, and a few possible vaccines that might prove effective after more testing.

But like USAMRIID, the NIH and CDC faced a lack of test subjects. Medical drugs are routinely tested in monkeys and chimpanzees, but nothing can be approved for widespread use in humans before a rigorous set of tests on subjects. And there weren't a lot of humans with Ebola walking around the suburbs of Washington, D.C., where the NIH is based, or Atlanta, the CDC's home turf.

That meant Favipiravir and other potential solutions could go through what is known as phase-one testing, designed to show whether a drug was actually safe for human consumption, but not later-stage tests aimed at deciding whether a drug is actually effective against a specific disease.

So when Favipiravir arrived in West Africa, NIH officials thought they could race through the testing process in a few months, something approaching record speed in the staid, glacial field of medical testing. But they still had to follow the same broad testing regimen any new drug undergoes: some patients would get the drug, a control group would not, and the mortality rates would be compared.

MSF officials were incensed. If a potential drug was available, they argued, every patient should get it, as soon as humanly possible. To withhold a potentially life-saving treatment, they believed, was a moral outrage.

"They interpreted research as not caring about the individual patient," said Anthony Fauci, director of the National Institute for Allergy and Infectious Diseases (NIAID) at the NIH. "They had no interest in answering in a definitive way the question of what [drugs] you would need for the next time" an outbreak swept through a community.

To Fauci, a wiry and compact epidemiologist with a thick New York accent and decades of experience with infectious disease, the impulse was understandable. Of course a treatment should be made available to anyone who might need it. But his experience gave him pause; over his career, he had seen even the most promising drugs harm patients.

Fauci has lasted longer in his post than most government officials. Appointed to head the NIAID in 1984, he arrived in the director's office just as the AIDS epidemic reached the height of the public imagination. During his three decades leading his institute, housed in a 1950s-era office building in desperate need of an upgrade on the NIH campuses just outside of Washington, Fauci's moments in the limelight have come during epidemics and outbreaks across the world, though much of his work has focused over the years on finding treatments for HIV and AIDS. So many of the drugs that made it to stage-two or stage-three testing, he said in an interview, were just as likely to harm a patient as to help.

Early tests of Favipiravir appeared to show promising results. The data showed that in Liberian villages where the drug was used, mortality rates were dramatically lower than in villages where the drug had not been distributed. According to MSF, that showed the drug was working and that it should be mass-produced and disseminated to all three countries. Fauci and his American colleagues looked beneath the toplines to draw a starkly different conclusion: The patients being treated with Favipiravir were surviving because the drug wasn't the only treatment they were receiving. Across the board, Favipiravir was administered in places where patients received much higher-quality medical treatment than in villages where the drug was not part of the treatment plan. Fauci and others concluded that the drug wasn't working at all; the mortality rates were coming down because Liberians and their nongovernmental organization partners were getting better at treating patients.

"It was the better medical care" that was bringing down mortality rates, Fauci concluded. "It likely had little to do with the drug."

But back in those early days, on the ground in Guinea and Liberia, the relief workers who had feuded so bitterly began to think the outbreak was following a similar pattern, running out of the fuel it needed to survive, and to thrive. WHO experts keeping tabs on the number of new cases saw those numbers tumble, from a dozen or more a day to a handful, then to zero. Between the end of April and the first week of May, just ten or so new cases were reported. A week went by with just two new cases in Guinea; that same week, doctors ruled out one possible case in Liberia, meaning the number of its infected actually fell, to twelve. For the rest of the month, Liberia would not record a single new case of Ebola.

The relief workers and virus hunters who had raced to the latest outbreak began to allow themselves the hope that maybe, just maybe, the outbreak would not be as disastrous as they feared. Arriving on May 5 in Lagos, Nigeria, for the World Economic Forum, USAID director Raj Shah detected a palpable sense of relief—the world might have just dodged a dangerous bullet.

"There was an early response that was geared to what people knew of an Ebola crisis in Africa," Shah explained later, drawing the typical bell curve that had defined earlier outbreaks on a lined legal pad. "It had a pattern and a strategy and a distribution, and we felt it was dissipating based on the trend lines."

Others saw the same hopeful trends. On May 6, 2014, Samaritan's Purse, a nongovernmental organization run by the American evangelist Franklin Graham, wrapped up its disaster response in Liberia. They had created a six-bed treatment center at a hospital in Monrovia, none of which had ever been filled.[6] The next day, Pierre Rollin, the CDC expert who had spent five and a half weeks in the hot zone, flew back to headquarters in Atlanta, ten days after his team had seen their last new case. MSF sent its staff in Liberia back to Guinea, where they could care for those still fighting the virus. Even the WHO began drawing down its operations.

In March, Piet deVries had begun holding initial meetings with friends at the Liberian Ministry of Health to plan a handover of Global Communities' water hygiene project after a decade on the ground. The handover halted as Global Communities pivoted to fight Ebola. Now, after spending a month and a half shipping supplies and resources to Liberia's northern rural counties, he too thought a corner had been turned. He headed back to Monrovia, to continue wrapping up his mission.

By May 22, Liberia had gone forty-two days without a new infection, a major milestone. Once infected with Ebola, the longest a patient can go without showing symptoms is twenty-one days. Once a country went the length of two consecutive incubation periods without a new infection, it would be deemed virus-free. In a news conference that day, Bernice Dahn, head of the Liberian Ministry of Health's Ebola response team, celebrated, cautiously, her country's accomplishment.[7]

"It looked like we had really beaten Ebola," deVries recalled later. "A very optimistic view of [the] circumstances would be that the virus was self-limiting and the epidemic was going to disappear," WHO's Chris Dye said.

Around the same time, Fabian Leendertz and his team of seventeen virus hunters were crossing the rickety bridge that connected Meliandou to the outside world. Contact tracers, working diligently to chart the virus from Sierra Leone and Liberia back across the border to its roots near Gueckedou, had settled on the small town atop a hill as the virus's likely source. Leendertz, an infectious diseases expert at the Robert Koch Institute in Berlin, hoped to solve the mystery of just where Ebola lives when it is not infecting humans. They knew whatever reservoir host passed the virus to little Emile had been in Meliandou, so they set off to search the village in hopes of identifying the culprit.

In the months since the outbreak began, Meliandou had undergone hard times. Neighboring villages had shunned its residents, and as many as a third of those who lived there had fled. Leendertz and his team, arriving in jeeps bumping along the single red dirt path, had to work overtime to win the villagers' trust.

"When those cars are coming with white people inside, they are normally to extract someone who has Ebola. But that was not our mission,"

Leendertz said. "They were really stigmatized from the other villages around. The good taxis would not go there anymore, and they were really isolated from the outside world."

Leendertz and his team visited Meliandou twice a day for ten days to win villagers' trust. Each time they left and returned, they had to brave the bridge, which outsiders had burned in hopes of isolating the village. It had been rebuilt, haphazardly, so Leendertz's team tested the untrustworthy logs positioned over the small river before each crossing. "For four times a day, we had to cross that stupid bridge," he recalled later.

Once the villagers trusted Leendertz and his team, the Europeans began asking questions: What kind of wildlife is around? There were no primates on which to feast, one manner of zoonotic transmission that had caused earlier outbreaks in Central Africa; the nearest rainforest, where monkeys and apes might live, was about three hours away. But there were bats, rodents, and a few other smaller species, all of which they set out to catch. One young man from the village helped the team cut branches into sticks they used to hold up bat-catching nets. It was important to Leendertz, and the anthropologist he had brought with him, to make Meliandou's remaining inhabitants aware that the Europeans valued their input, their advice, and their theories.

The team asked about hollowed out trees, where a colony of bats might live. Grudgingly, villagers told them about one such tree, a few meters from the outer ring of homes. They had burned it just days before, when Guinea's government told villagers that bush meat was to be avoided.

The tree had been home to a colony of bats, and after Emile got sick, it had become a source of suspicion. Both of those facts were important clues to Leendertz's team. While no one has ever isolated live Ebola virus in bats, scientists strongly suspect certain species of the flying mammals are Ebola's reservoir host. They cannot say it without rigorous scientific proof, but few virologists and epidemiologists think something other than a bat might be harboring Ebola in between human outbreaks.

After burning the tree, villagers had collected enough dead animals to fill an entire rice bag with corpses. And while the animals were gone, Leendertz was able to collect soil from nearby, which contained enough genetic material to allow him to identify the species of bat that inhabited the tree—Angolan free-tailed bats, *Mops condylurus*, an animal with a massive range stretching from Liberia to Somalia all the way to South Africa. It was not enough to prove that the insect- and fruit-eating bats were responsible for Emile's illness, but their presence was a telling clue.

About an hour outside of Monrovia, Randy Schoepp began thinking about home. After almost a decade spent traveling between his home in Frederick, Maryland, and Sierra Leone to study Lassa fever, Schoepp's team had re-deployed to a small HIV clinic, where they converted several rooms into a highly secure testing lab. To stay clear of the technicians in the rest of the clinic, Schoepp took over a four-room suite on the second floor, in the very back, far enough away, he hoped, to avoid exposing anyone to blood samples that might be teeming with the virus.

In those early days, few organizations had the capability to test blood samples for the Ebola virus; Schoepp, using a hugely expensive device about the size and shape of a large coffee machine, could. Carefully, Schoepp's team trained five Liberians in the delicate art of operating in level-four conditions, burdened by hefty space suits that rang with the deafening tone of air being pumped in. Encumbered as they were, the technicians learned to process a potentially infected blood sample, pulling out and isolating RNA, then binding it to one of the assays that would allow the coffee pot machine to show whether Ebola was present.

But by the time he had arrived, Schoepp wondered if he was too late. After a month in the hot zone, Schoepp's team had received thirteen samples to test. They were all negative, free of the virus.

"Maybe we missed it. Maybe this was the end of it," Schoepp thought.

Schoepp boarded a commercial airliner, connected in Europe, and landed at Washington's Dulles International Airport, still about an hour from his home near Fort Detrick. He had barely cleared customs when a text message made his phone vibrate. It was one of the Liberian technicians with an urgent message: You need to come back. Something has happened.

The bad luck of the early phase of the outbreak was that the Ebola virus had jumped an international border, from Guinea to Liberia. The miracle was that it had not jumped other borders, into Sierra Leone or Côte d'Ivoire, two neighboring nations where tribal connections were thicker than any relationship with far-off national governments.

But on May 23, just a day after Liberia had been deemed free of the virus, a pregnant woman arrived at the government-run hospital in Kenema, Sierra Leone, the very hospital where Schoepp's team and Garry's team had conducted their Lassa tests. She showed signs of being sick.

Robert Garry had been traveling to Sierra Leone for ten years, ever since Tulane won an NIH grant to work on Lassa fever in 2005. Over that time, the trip from Freetown to Kenema had been cut from a grueling twelve-hour slog over roads no wider than an alley to a relatively easy three-hour trip, over more modern roads built by Chinese and Italian investors. Garry's hunch had been that previous work he had done, developing tests to seek out the HIV virus, would apply to Lassa. In Kenema, the heart of Lassa's endemic territory, Garry's tests had been so successful that they had branched out and begun testing assays that would identify another hemorrhagic fever, Ebola.

When the young pregnant woman with flu-like symptoms showed up, the head of Kenema's Lassa unit, Dr. Sheik Umar Khan, knew he might be looking at his country's first Ebola case; after all, the hospital is just a few miles from the border with Liberia, where the disease had only just been stamped out, and a short drive from the border with Guinea, where cases were still present. Khan had years of experience with hemorrhagic fevers himself, and he knew what to do. He donned a full-body protective suit, a head covering made of strong white Tyvek fabric, a breathing mask, a face shield, goggles, and two pairs of surgical gloves. Over that, he added a pair of rubber gloves, high rubber boots, and a plastic apron.

Khan drew the woman's blood, then sent it to Schoepp's old lab for testing. When the results came back positive the next day, he placed the woman in isolation. Though she lost the baby, miraculously, Sierra Leone's first Ebola victim recovered.

Virus trackers raced to the scene to interview the woman. They had to know: Where had she come from? Where might she have contracted the virus? What they learned was shocking. The patient had attended a funeral for a local healer, a woman who said her traditional remedies and incantations, and the snakes she placed on the bodies of the sick, could cure the mystery disease raging through the Forest Region. The healer had tended to many Ebola patients, and after so much contact, she too fell ill. On April 8, the healer died.

Hundreds of mourners had participated in her funeral across the border, in a predominantly Muslim district of Liberia. The village where she had died was just a few hours from Kenema, over bumpy roads, but close enough that doctors knew they could expect a wave of new cases. A subsequent investigation traced an incredible 365 deaths from Ebola to the faith healer's funeral; the first 13 Ebola victims in Sierra Leone had all attended her funeral.[8]

But the doctors were optimistic that they could stem the tide, if they worked quickly and aggressively to track new cases. Garry sent his two teams of four investigators each north to the Kailahun District, and the town of Koindu, just across the border from the outbreak's epicenter, in their old but rugged vehicles.

The reports those teams sent back quickly deprived Garry of any hope that the virus had been contained. The investigators found whole villages that looked like something out of a zombie movie. The villages were decimated, bodies lying in the streets, the sick and dying were everywhere. One team found a home containing six dead bodies.

Soon, some of those infected followed the pregnant woman to Kenema. Their instincts were right; the hospital was the only facility in West Africa with a dedicated isolation ward, albeit one initially designed to treat patients with Lassa fever.

"The cases just started to come. It was apparent there had been a lot more cases up there," Garry said.

But a hospital in West Africa, even one equipped with a hemorrhagic fever isolation ward, is hardly what Westerners would consider a suitable medical facility. "We wouldn't even call it a hospital," Schoepp recalled of his old office. "We would call it a group of sheds that happen to have some very poor medical equipment."

Kenema's hospital had enough beds to handle about two hundred patients. It was made up of low cinderblock buildings, all of which were just one-story tall. The various wards—a maternity ward, separate wards for treating men and women, a converted administrative building that served as the Lassa ward—were spread out across the small campus, fenced in on all sides. Construction was begun on a new, more modern Lassa ward, which would house forty-four beds, three times the size of the current unit. That current unit was tiny; it held only seven beds, enough space for fourteen patients, if they shared beds.

Almost immediately, the hospital was overwhelmed. WHO statistics tell the sterilized story: A report on May 27 shows one confirmed case of Ebola, the pregnant woman. A report from the next day, May 28, shows sixteen cases—more than the total outbreak so far in Liberia. Five days later, there were fifty cases, then eighty-one in another three days, most of them at Kenema. The numbers do nothing to convey the sorrow, the horror, of a hospital ill-equipped to handle the onslaught. Patients soon lined the hallways, moaning in pain and delirium into the night. Without the same protective measures Khan had taken, nurses began to fall ill. Within just a few weeks, twelve had died.

Cases soon popped up in Kailahun, a district capital near the intersection of Sierra Leone, Guinea, and Liberia. Then the first resident of Freetown, Sierra Leone's capital city, population nearly a million, showed symptoms. Across the border, new patients were falling ill in Guinea, and then in Liberia. In the final week of May, the number of cases in Guinea shot from 258 to 281. By the first week of June, the case count rose to 344.

In Liberia, cases began rising, too. A few weeks after he had returned to Monrovia, deVries received a call from Tamba Boima, a Liberian Ministry of Health official he counted as a close friend. Boima had traveled north, to Lofa County, on the border with Guinea. Ebola had reemerged in Voinjama, Lofa's capital, a city of 270,000.

"You've got to come back," Boima told deVries. "We need to do another [public education] program."

The neat bell curve that was supposed to map out Ebola's decline was suddenly trending back upward. Something had happened; even as Liberia was declared virus-free, even as Guinea's trajectory looked so promising, someone—more accurately, everyone—had missed a sign. The virus hunters who had gone home in early May now turned around, packed their bags once again, and boarded flights back to a much more complicated situation than they had left behind.

Ebola had found new fuel.

FIVE

Roaring Back

THE FAMILIAR CURVE THAT showed the Ebola outbreak subsiding in May 2014 allowed epidemiologists and virologists the chance to breathe, to rotate home and see families after a harrowing month. It allowed the world to turn its attention to the seemingly endless crises elsewhere: the annexation of Crimea by Russian forces, the perilous debt crisis that threatened Greece, and with it the future of the eurozone, the devastating civil war in Syria, and the growing threat of a particularly aggressive jihadist group that, by the end of June, would declare itself the Islamic State, all vying for space among the headlines.

But the health workers who had been closest to their colleagues and friends in Guinea, Liberia, and Sierra Leone began to hear reports in increasing numbers that the downward trend in Ebola cases was reversing itself. The disease was once again on the march.

Soon, doctors who had remained behind or rotated in to take their own shifts were overwhelmed. It was like being in a giant whack-a-mole game, where the moles popped up too fast. In late May and early June, new cases emerged in Conakry, Guinea's capital; in Telimele, in central Guinea; and in the tiny town of Boffa, along one of Guinea's main highways north of the capital. In the Forest Region, fifteen new cases emerged in the final week of May.

"There was an impression that [Ebola] had been contained," said Amy Pope, President Obama's deputy national security adviser who would be intimately involved in the American response. "So then when it became clear that there was a pretty significant outbreak in the Forest Region, it kind of caught everybody by surprise."

On his way home to New Orleans in early June, Robert Garry stopped in Washington to raise the alarm. A soft-spoken man with a bushy mustache, Garry hunches over; he has a tendency to chuckle in uncomfortable situations. This situation was less uncomfortable than it was urgent: the outbreak was rebounding.

Garry found a receptive audience at the National Institutes of Health (NIH), where several of his longtime colleagues shared his anxiety. But his reception at other federal departments—the Department of Health and Human Services, the State Department, the United States Agency for International Development (USAID)—was less accommodating. The humanitarian experts Garry met with were polite, though they made clear they did not share his urgency. Several of those experts told him that the World Health Organization (WHO) was insisting everything was still under control.

Garry wondered where WHO was getting its information. In June, a single WHO doctor, Tom Fletcher, had showed up at the Kenema hospital. He told Garry he had taken the initiative to travel to West Africa on his own; his agency had not sent him.

The challenge health workers faced was evident hundreds of miles to the east, where Harisson Sakilla worked as a principal at a mission school in Liberia's Foya district, at the crossroads where all three countries meet. In late May, according to a UNICEF diary, the thirty-nine-year-old got word that his mother had fallen ill at her home in Kpondu, across the border in Sierra Leone. Assuming she had malaria or some other common disease, he walked two hours down a dirt path to care for her. Finding her too weak to seek treatment on her own, Sakilla took a canoe across the Makona River into Guinea to another village where he could buy drugs. Within a single day, one man had set foot in all three countries, without once encountering anything resembling a border control operation.

Sakilla cared for his mother for three more days, as she alternately writhed in delirium or sat, glassy-eyed and nearly comatose. As she lay close to death, Sakilla returned to his own village in Liberia to buy the material in which she would be buried. At her funeral, Sakilla watched as his mother's body was washed, clothed, and wrapped for burial. He may have been one of the dozens who kissed her body, a traditional lament in West African funerals. For three more days, he and his relatives grieved over their loss.

On the fourth day, on his walk home, he felt ill. His joints were weak, his body wracked by fever. He had diarrhea, and a walk that ordinarily took two hours stretched to an agonizing four. Days later, Sakilla went to a new Ebola Treatment Center in Foya, run by Médecins Sans Frontières (MSF), where he was the first patient to be admitted. After more than a month of treatment, at times teetering between life and death, watching those around him carted in on stretchers and out in body bags, Sakilla walked out with a certificate issued by Samaritan's Purse showing he was free of the disease. As he walked back to his home, his wife ran down the dirt path outside their house, shrieking with joy. Harisson embraced his six children; their father had survived.[1]

But Sakilla's story was rare. After his mother died and as he lay fighting for his own life in the treatment center in Foya, Harisson had lost his father, his sister, his older brother, a niece, and the niece's daughter.[2] The pattern repeated again and again across all three countries, while the world was otherwise distracted.

By the time Randy Schoepp arrived back at the HIV diagnostics clinic outside Monrovia, he could plainly see that the atmosphere was different. After the Liberian technician had texted him to ask him to return, Schoepp had spent only a week back home, before reboarding a flight bound first for Europe, then for Monrovia.

On his first deployment to Liberia, the 13 samples Schoepp had tested had come back negative. When he returned, almost all tested positive. And at the rate at which samples were arriving at the lab, the team began working furiously, around the clock, just to keep pace. First they were processing 15 to 20 samples a day, then 30 or 45. By the late summer, they reached a capacity of 120 or more every day. The samples arrived at all hours of the day and night, in boxes packed in delivery trucks or on the backs of motorcycles. They were handed off to a technician on the ground floor of the two-story facility, then taken upstairs to the windowless, oppressively hot four-room suite where diagnostics tests could be run, as far away from everyone else in the building as the technicians could hide themselves.

The technicians, dressed in head-to-toe personal protection equipment, would carefully unwrap the package in what virus hunters call a "gray" room, a space where one had to assume that Ebola was present, and therefore had to take precautions when entering and exiting. The technicians would remove any paper that had come along with the sample—patient details like names, ages, genders, treatment center locations—and disinfect the paper. The sample itself was taken next door, to an extraction room, the dirtiest room, where one was most likely to encounter Ebola, in the suite. Transferred to a glass tube, the sample would then proceed to a third room, where it would be combined with the assay, the chemical compound designed to show whether Ebola was present. The assay had come from another room, the fourth and cleanest—most likely to be Ebola-free—in the suite.

In the third room, Schoepp stared at the computer screen for hours on end, waiting for each result to come back. Seemingly every sample revealed the same answer: Positive. Positive. Positive.

As so many cases emerged, virtual death sentences for those infected, Schoepp thought back to an episode of MASH, in which one of the American doctors serving in Korea is asked whether he sees the faces of the men he treats. No, the doctor replies, he just sees a blur. Anything more would be too much for one soul to take. Schoepp searched for his own coping mechanisms.

Even then, relief was scarce. In many instances, a well-organized medical response will code patients, assigning them numbers to avoid confusion that might come with keeping track of often-similar names. But in Liberia, the samples that crossed Schoepp's desk were attached to actual names and the villages where they were being treated. In the course of those chaotic weeks, from his vantage point sometimes hundreds of miles away, Schoepp watched entire families, entire clans, entire villages come down with Ebola. One family in particular stuck with him: it was a family of seven, from a predominantly Muslim village in northern Liberia, that had attended a funeral. Their samples arrived together: six of the seven tested positive. The only one that turned up negative was the youngest child, five years old, who had been too young to take part in the funeral rites.

The light cycler Schoepp and his team relied on for diagnostics, the one that resembles a large coffeemaker, would test thirty-two samples at a time, contained in glass tubes. As the number of samples increased, Schoepp began asking, with greater and greater urgency, for upgraded equipment. The light cycler used technology that was more than a decade old. He wanted an AB 7500, a much more advanced machine that looks like a large, high-speed business printer (it is, in fact, quite a bit more expensive than a high-speed business printer). That machine could test ninety-six samples at a time, using a plastic tray about the size of an index card rather than glass tubes. Schoepp joked later, ruefully, almost relieved, that the presence of glass in a highly secure containment laboratory is not exactly ideal. It took weeks for the notoriously slow Pentagon procurement process to work, but when the new machine arrived, the diagnostic lab's capacity for testing samples skyrocketed.

The tests on both machines would take hours to complete. In the light cycler, the tubes spun at high velocity, separating RNA from the blood sample and combining it with the assay. The AB 7500 dripped the assay into each space on its tray of ninety-six divots. As each machine recorded flashes of fluorescence, the indication that the assay had found its target and that a sample had Ebola, it would spit out its results in the form of a line graph on a laptop sitting nearby. The brighter the flash, the more certain Schoepp could be that Ebola was present; if a sample produced a line on the graph that peaked over a certain threshold, the patient had the virus.

In the movies, the testing process is clear and straightforward: sample goes in, computer spits out a clear result, and someone is either sick or well. In the sweltering heat of the Liberian rainy season, an ocean away from the carefully controlled laboratories of the U.S. Army Medical Research Institute for Infectious Diseases (USAMRIID), the testing process is far more fraught, and far less conclusive. The lines on the graph that were supposed to be so neatly logarithmic were instead choppy, and sometimes inconclusive. Schoepp feared the prospect of making a mistake and misdiagnosing a patient: tell an infected person they do not have the disease, and they will return home to infect their family and friends. Tell someone without the disease that they are infected, and they will enter an Ebola ward, where they are almost certain to catch Ebola, and then overwhelmingly likely to die.

Some samples were indeterminate. Others showed the presence of Ebola, but in patients who appeared to be getting better. Doctors in overcrowded Ebola treatment centers needed those beds for new patients who were suffering more, but Schoepp could not guarantee those patients were virus-free.

Each night, exhausted after hours and hours in oppressively humid personal protection equipment, the USAMRIID team would leave the converted HIV clinic to return to their rooms in an upscale corporate resort where the choicest rooms faced the beach and the Atlantic Ocean. By day, Schoepp worried that one of his technicians might become ill. By night, he worried that they might not make it back to the resort alive because the roads were so treacherous. There were no streetlights, and people and animals crossing the road were a constant danger. Every minor rise could be hiding a stalled truck, which barely bothered to pull off to the side as drivers worked without hazard lights to make their repairs. Even during daylight hours, driving in Liberia is different, and turn signals routinely go unemployed. The Liberians driving the team back and forth, trained in evasive driving techniques by American diplomatic security personnel based at the U.S. embassy, narrowly avoided countless accidents.

Back at the resort, the mental strain weighed on the diagnosticians. After spending their first deployment in fancy rooms overlooking the beach, slowly, one by one, they moved to rooms closer to the lobby; the sound of the ocean contrasted with their inability to unwind became maddening. In three long deployments, Schoepp found time to take a brief walk on the beach just twice.

At the same time, technicians and health workers in other parts of the HIV clinic were falling ill, and those who did not were still touched by the disease: they would return home at night to communities and neighborhoods ravaged by Ebola. None of Schoepp's Liberian technicians ever fell ill, but several had family members who got sick. The technicians would bring in their own samples to be tested. Schoepp, alarmed, had to tell them to stop: He couldn't stand to see his colleagues risk their own lives by drawing blood from someone who could be ill.

Back at the hospital in Kenema, where Khan and his team were so experienced in diagnosing and treating Lassa, the Sierra Leonean doctors and nurses set the stage for a new attack on Ebola, one that would require genetically sequencing the disease to discover its secrets—and, potentially, its vulnerabilities. Khan and Pardis Sabeti, a biology professor at Harvard, collected samples of Ebola-infected blood left over after other samples were sent to the diagnostics labs. They ended up with samples from forty-nine individuals who were either infected or suspected to be infected; those samples, after being sterilized with chemicals to ensure the virus was dead, traveled by DHL Express to Sabeti's lab at Harvard. The package arrived on June 4; Stephen Gire, one of Sabeti's fellow researchers, had to open the box with his car keys because he had forgotten to bring a knife.[3]

The alarming death rates among West African health-care workers spooked those Westerners who had arrived to help. By the time Joe Woodring arrived in Liberia for his first deployment, it was clear the efforts to diminish the presence of Ebola were long gone—no one entered or left any building of significance without washing their hands in chlorine solution. Men armed with handheld devices to measure body temperature were positioned everywhere, checking for fever. No one shook hands; some greeted each other by touching elbows, but even that sterile contact made others nervous.

Woodring, a native of the Philadelphia area, was deployed as a senior medical specialist by the Centers for Disease Control and Prevention (CDC). He stepped into an atmosphere of strict rules designed to keep health-care workers safe, and he soon found himself developing what was effectively a four-foot bubble, staying far enough away from anyone who might possibly be infected, and even those who had contact with the potentially infected. Soon, subtly, without noticing it himself, Woodring began positioning himself upwind of anyone who had even the slightest cough.

When, on occasion, Woodring had to break the bubble, a shiver of terror ran up his spine. Once in a while, when paying for lunch, he might make inadvertent contact with a waiter or cashier. They would freeze, meet each other's eyes in a moment of panic, and think to themselves: "Oh, shit."

The safety precautions extended to those he worked with most closely. After leaving Liberia at the end of his first deployment, Woodring said goodbye to his colleague, a partner with whom he had spent a month in the hot zone. The two men realized that, for the entire month, they had never made physical contact—no handshake, no pat on the back, no grab of the arm. Standing in the bustling terminal of the Brussels airport, minutes before catching connecting flights home, the two men embraced.

In those early weeks of June, many of the scientists who had breathed sighs of relief just a month earlier were returning in force. New Ebola treatment centers opened around all three countries: MSF's facility opened in Foya in early June; another MSF facility would open in Kailahun, in Sierra Leone, three weeks later. A nongovernmental organization called Eternal Love Winning Africa—ELWA for short—opened its first facility in Monrovia, sandwiched between a major highway and the Atlantic Ocean, a few blocks from the Sugarcane Beach Lounge. There, a Samaritan's Purse doctor named Kent Brantley, who had served as a missionary physician in Liberia since the previous October, welcomed the first patient on June 11.

The mystery over the sudden influx of new cases demonstrated the underlying problem that world health officials had from the beginning. Though they believed they had accurately tracked the number of people who were sick and dying, it became clear that the estimates had entirely missed new outbreaks in places like the Forest Region and in rural counties where international borders meant nothing, where tribal connections ran deep, and where suspicion of national governments was pervasive. The number of cases had never gone down; the infected patients had so distrusted the men in moon suits that they simply hid, preferring traditional treatments from shamans and snakes to a seemingly guaranteed death in a harsh and desolate treatment center.

The need to accurately track and positively identify those who have been in contact with someone who is sick is as critical a tool in outbreak response as actually treating a patient. That practice, known as contact tracing, is relatively easy when an outbreak takes place in the remote forests of the Congo, where an entire village and its contacts may number no more than a few hundred. But in Conakry, Freetown, and Monrovia, cities of hundreds of thousands of people, and in highly mobile rural areas, tracking down complex social webs is frighteningly challenging, whether in slums or far-flung villages. Making matters more complicated were tribal suspicions and customs, which created a tough-to-navigate social network worthy of volumes of anthropological and cultural research.

The best contact tracers in this world of uncertainty were those who already knew the contours of the deeply woven relationships. The best contact tracers were people like Mosoka Fallah.

Fallah is a big man in his mid-forties. His friends describe him as a man with a loud laugh and a kind face. He is a study in perhaps the starkest socioeconomic contrast that could possibly exist. Raised in Monrovia slums with names like West Point and Chicken Soup Factory, he won a scholarship to study at Harvard, where he became an epidemiologist and immunologist. His international connections allowed him to speak comfortably before donors and officials at the world's most important nongovernmental organizations, to his own government ministers, and to well-placed officials in the United States and Europe. He was equally comfortable in Monrovia, speaking to a mother living in a ramshackle hodgepodge of corrugated iron and wood, whose son might have Ebola.

As Ebola raged around him, Fallah led contact tracing teams into the neighborhoods where he had grown up. His teams found countless Ebola victims, and countless more potential cases. But sometimes, as in the case with the young mother, Fallah had to employ a special touch.

The mother lived in West Point, one of Liberia's impoverished slums. She had refused to tell any of Fallah's investigators, who arrived in their frightening space suits, where her eight-year-old child had gone. The boy had come into contact with a neighbor who had Ebola, putting him at high risk for catching the disease. But as curious neighbors gathered around the men in space suits, the mother's anxiety rose: if her child had Ebola, the family would be shunned, the stigma of the virus forcing them out of their homes.

The next day, Fallah arrived in the slums, alone. He parked his car far away from the mother's home, so the neighbors would not see; all he brought with him was lunch. While they ate, they talked. The mother said her son's father was abusive, and rarely present. When he did appear, he would take his son out. If his mother objected, she was beaten.

She had already taken the risk of reporting her son's contact with an Ebola patient, the same report she denied making the next day. The boy's father had come for one of his occasional visits; if he knew the boy's mother had included their son on the Ebola contact list, the beating would be especially severe. The only way she could find her son, the mother told Fallah, was to hire a motorbike taxi. But she had no money.

Fallah dug into his pocket and produced a crisp bill. The woman recoiled—no one in the slums had a crisp bill. If the money in her pocket weren't dirty and soiled, her neighbors would know something was amiss. Fallah crinkled the bill, rubbed it on his clothes, anything to give it a well-worn look. Still, the mother rejected his gift. Finally, Fallah walked to a nearby market, where he bought something small, exchanging his newer bill for the old, ratty currency that circulated in the slums. The mother sped off on the back of a taxi. The next day, Fallah's team found her son back in his mother's home.

"This is not data. This is rapport. This is the ability to speak to a vulnerable woman," said Hans Rosling, an internationally recognized Swedish epidemiologist who knew Fallah well and who related the story. "Anthropology is as important as statistics. Understanding the individual is as important as counting them."

"Let them see you as part of them," Fallah told an alumni magazine at his alma mater, Harvard's T. H. Chan School of Public Health. "When I entered West Point, I never stayed in my car. I got out and I walked and I met the leaders. I walked with them in the houses and in between the houses. I never touched them—it was an epidemic, and I kept my distance. But I wasn't bringing this big Harvard degree to them. I wasn't telling them that I knew it all. I let the leaders make decisions and I guided them and followed them."[4]

More Fallahs were racing back from their homes overseas. On June 21, MSF tried to grab the world's attention: The epidemic, they said, had spiraled "out of control." By the time MSF opened their thirty-two-bed facility in Kailahun five days later, they were immediately overwhelmed. The facility eventually grew to sixty-five beds to accommodate as many of the sick as they could.

Back in the United States, senior health officials were beginning to hear alarming reports from their own people. Cliff Lane, a researcher at the U.S. Institute of Allergy and Infectious Diseases, returned from a visit to Liberia, where he had been setting up a trial of a new vaccine. Briefing his boss, Anthony Fauci, Lane called the outbreak a "catastrophe." Tom Frieden, the director of the CDC, told Fauci much the same thing. But even the CDC acknowledged later it had not taken proper heed of MSF's warning, and of the increasingly troubling reports from the field.

"We got it wrong, as did a lot of people, when we thought the outbreak was contained," Frieden said later. "Within a couple of weeks, we realized, Woah, [the MSF warnings] were completely right. This is different. We've never seen anything like this before. This is urban Ebola."

Still, the World Health Organization hesitated. On June 15, WHO sent its first monitors into Sierra Leone, alarmed by a rapid spike in new cases. The next month, it established a regional coordinating center in Guinea. Fauci and Frieden in the United States, and virtually every other group on the ground in West Africa, watched with increasing alarm as WHO resisted making a formal declaration of an emergency. That declaration would get the world's attention, allow more resources to flow into West Africa, and stanch the damage before hundreds, maybe thousands, more were infected.

"When the cases were on their way up, had not yet peaked, it was very, very clear to Tom and I . . . that the WHO was not recognizing the seriousness of this," Fauci later recalled.

The WHO's July 2 report showed that 413 people had been infected in Guinea, 107 in Liberia, and 239 in Sierra Leone, almost certainly just a fraction of the real number that had come down with the disease. The mortality rate stood north of 60 percent; in Guinea, 75 percent of those who contracted Ebola had died.

"The world writ large missed the uptick in mid-June to late July," said Rajiv Shah, head of USAID.

S I X

Death of a Hero

ALMOST EVERY TOP EPIDEMIOLOGIST and virologist streaming into West
Africa already knew Sheik Umar Khan. For a decade, Khan had run the
region's only medical ward dedicated to treating and researching Lassa fever,
at Sierra Leone's Kenema Government Hospital about 190 miles from Freetown. His big, gregarious smile, teeth exposed, erupted at the sight of friends
and colleagues; even in a community of energetic professionals known for
pushing themselves to and beyond their physical limits, Khan developed
a reputation for his enthusiasm. He would end many long days with
colleagues—Randy Schoepp, the U.S. Army Medical Research Institute for
Infectious Diseases (USAMRIID) diagnostician who worked in the Lassa
ward, and Robert Garry, the Tulane epidemiologist—over beers, excitedly
discussing their progress and what they could investigate next. In early May,
Garry and Khan had traveled to a conference in Nigeria; they spent eight
hours at Freetown's airport during a flight delay, talking.

Now, as May turned to June, Khan found himself on the front lines in
the battle to contain another hemorrhagic fever, Ebola.

Friends say Khan was driven by a deep desire to improve himself—just
weeks before the outbreak came to Sierra Leone, he had completed a training course to improve his knowledge of clinical medicine, and he was

scheduled to take a sabbatical at Harvard, to help map the genomes of hemorrhagic fevers.

He was also driven by an urge to improve his country, scarred as it had been by civil wars. He had fled into exile in neighboring Guinea three times during the 1990s, when rebels rose up and captured Freetown. Several of his siblings moved to the United States and urged him to follow; he refused, and he was one of the first to return to the capital when British troops forced rebels out.

Khan had developed his fascination with medicine at an early age. One of ten children of a school headmaster in Lungi, just outside Freetown, he befriended the children of a nearby couple who ran a clinic for expectant mothers. Just a few years after earning his medical degree, at the age of twenty-nine, Khan leaped at the chance to take over Kenema's Lassa ward, when his predecessor, Aniru Conteh, died after getting infected through an accidental needle prick.

Khan quickly became a staple in Kenema, where he maintained a private practice treating patients alongside his duties in the Lassa ward. He could be found at the Capitol, a hotel and restaurant near the hospital, watching his favorite team, AC Milan, play soccer on the satellite television. Some patrons might have been alarmed to see him celebrate goals by ripping off his shirt and waving it over his head.[1] His dedication to the hospital cost him his marriage to a childhood sweetheart, who moved to London.

And when Ebola arrived, perhaps no medical professional in all of Sierra Leone was better prepared. Khan knew Ebola was lurking in the nearby jungles, and he took precautions to protect himself; he saw the first suspected patient, the young pregnant woman, while decked out in full personal protection equipment. Her blood test came back negative for Lassa, but it was clear the young woman was suffering from a hemorrhagic fever.

"We were concerned that cases that were testing negative for Lassa fever . . . are presenting as acute viral illnesses," Khan told an interviewer of those early days. "What else could it be?"[2]

The Kenema Government Hospital's Lassa ward had been established first in the 1970s. In 2005, just after Khan took over, it had helped develop the first diagnostic test for Lassa, and in 2014 it had won a major grant from the U.S. Navy to build a new ward, one with forty-four beds and critical modern features like air conditioning, to protect doctors at risk of over-heating in sweltering space suits; tiled floor; and a modern drainage system. (Construction on the new ward paused during the outbreak as workers fled the disease, and the hospital.)[3] The Lassa ward was staffed by nurses who had suffered from, but survived, the hemorrhagic fever, which made them immune to catching the disease a second time.

But Kenema remained far below the standards of a traditional Western hospital. It was, in Schoepp's description, little more than a series of shacks, full of outdated medical equipment. Its roof was made of corrugated tin, its beds resembling flat beach chairs with slats, through which diarrhea and blood would ooze. Twisted wires held the metal walls together. In June, one of the walls collapsed; Khan ordered it rebuilt, with lower ceilings so it would be more stable.[4] When nurses ran low on supplies, they would wash out pairs of latex gloves, only meant to be used once, and leave them in the hot African sun to dry.

As possible Ebola cases mounted, even the relatively well-prepared hospital was quickly overwhelmed. Patients would arrive in a big white canvas tent, known as the annex, to have their blood drawn and wait for their diagnosis. Confirmed cases would be taken to Ward A, which could accommodate about thirty patients in its eight rooms. As those beds filled, patients were taken to a hastily constructed Ward B. Technicians in personal protection equipment would remove dead bodies to a makeshift morgue, a small shed behind Ward A, where they were stacked like cords of wood. The pile grew so high in June that some would tumble off the top, obstructing walkways.

Soon Garry's team of investigators found themselves working closer and closer to home, tracking contacts in Kenema itself. The teams counted every case they could, even those for whom they did not have space in the hospital. They traced contacts. They watched their own community get sick. They spent their days off, Garry recalled quietly a year later, "going to funerals."

But Khan made a point of showing compassion when he could. On the rare occasion that a patient was able to leave the hospital after fighting off the disease, Khan would hug them, in public, to show that survival was possible.

"These are people I embrace myself on the day of discharge, because don't forget the stigma about Ebola," he told a local newspaper.[5] "With some people, you have to give them certificates so that by the time they return to their villages people will understand that they are no more suffering from the disease and they are free to interact with the population. . . . I embrace them to, of course, tell the public that yes, this is the situation."

Those optimistic moments were few, and rapidly becoming fewer. Khan worked ten-hour days, then twelve, then seemingly nonstop, caring for patients. His office, where he dressed in his own personal protection gear, was nothing more than a trailer positioned next to the isolation wards. Its mirror, in which he checked for cuts or tears, was "the policeman," he said—his own way to ease his mind before entering the hot zone. Still, he was aware of the risks he was taking. He told his interviewer:

Of course, I am afraid for my life, because I must say I cherish my life. And if you are afraid of it you will take the maximum precautions, which I am doing. If you neglect . . . then you will ignore most of these personal protective equipment [PPE] and you wouldn't do things correctly. So having that in the back of my mind I make sure whenever I am going into the isolation unit I make sure that I am in full PPE.

Khan's family begged him to leave, like so many other doctors had. Once again, Khan said he would stay.

"If I refuse to treat [my patients], who would treat me?" he asked his sister.[6]

He repeatedly demanded that his nurses, so many of whom were like family to him, take the same precautions—dress in head-to-toe personal protection equipment, wash repeatedly with chlorine solution. When the outbreak moved into Sierra Leone, Robert Garry arrived with nine trunks, filled until bulging with gloves, masks, and Tyvek suits, enough gear for nine hundred clothing changes.

Soon, those clothing changes began to run out. By early July, Khan spent hours a day e-mailing colleagues, former classmates, and every American official he could remember, begging for supplies. They needed chlorine, gloves, goggles, protective suits, and salts to fight the dehydration that ultimately killed so many Ebola patients. He asked for 3,000 adult-sized body bags, and 2,000 small enough for children.[7]

But not every nurse took those precautions seriously. Some wore shoes from home into the isolation wards, then sprayed them down with hoses before going home. Khan himself was seen lifting his goggles inside the isolation ward to clear condensation that formed on the lenses.

There were other holes in security, too: When the chief of a local tribe arrived at a private ward on the hospital's campus, he infected the nurse who treated him. That nurse was pregnant; when she fell ill, four other nurses from Khan's ward helped induce labor to deliver her stillborn baby. It was a risky procedure, both for the woman and her nurse colleagues, but they knew it was the only chance they had to save her life. Blood was everywhere.[8] All four nurses who tended to the young woman got sick themselves.

One of those nurses was Mbalu Fonnie, the hospital's head nurse. Mbalu was a pillar in her community; many had mourned alongside her the year before when her husband, who headed Kenema Government Hospital's outreach team, had died of liver cancer. She was held in such high regard, with such a close relationship to the director, that Khan called her Mom.

By the time she was infected, Kenema was overrun, with more than seventy patients in treatment or isolation. Instead of placing her in the ward with those patients, Khan broke protocol to place her in a private room in the observation wing. It hardly mattered—virtually every sample taken from a patient in the observation wing was coming back positive anyway. Khan was working almost alone; the other doctors at the hospital had all fled, or died.

Security at the hospital was nonexistent. It was left unguarded, and some patients, either desperate to save themselves or delirious from the disease raging inside them, simply got up and left. When Fonnie fell ill, a vigil held in her honor outside the hospital rippled, then roared with rumors that she had died. The crowd became angry and threatened to storm the hospital. Though the police were summoned, there wasn't much they could do. The crowd was stilled only by Khan himself, alone, clearly near the edge of his capacity.

"My nurses are dead," Khan told the crowd. "And I don't know if I'm already infected or not."[9]

A few days later, Khan and his closest friend, a nurse named Alex Moig-boi, walked out of Ward A, after hours in the dripping heat. They undressed, raised their arms to be sprayed by chlorine solution. Moigboi turned to Khan to confess: He wasn't feeling well. He had treated the young pregnant nurse a few weeks earlier. Without thinking, out of pure instinct, Khan reached for Alex's eyes for a quick look, making skin-to-skin contact.[10]

Moigboi's test came back positive. On July 19, the day Moigboi died, Khan returned home feeling more exhausted than usual. He told his assistant he was worried. At a staff meeting at the hospital that day, several people noticed he appeared unwell. The fever came back that afternoon, and so did a headache. On Sunday, July 20, Khan woke up too sick to work. He managed to get himself to the hospital, where his own blood was tested. The tests came back negative. The same day, Fonnie succumbed.

On Tuesday, Khan's condition had not improved. Technicians drew more blood and ran a second test. Khan tried to rest at home, but hours later the district medical officer showed up—these tests had come back positive. Khan's blood was filling with the Ebola virus.

Khan and the medical officer considered their options, but they both decided the least palatable would be to check Khan in to his own hospital. Morale was already low, and watching their ace doctor, their national hero, fight for his life could destroy what little of it was left. The better option was to transfer Khan to the Médecins Sans Frontières (MSF) Ebola treatment center in Kailahun, seventy-five miles away. Khan climbed into an ambulance for a grueling, bumpy five-hour ride through a torrential monsoon.

The MSF facility in Kailahun was more modern than the Kenema Government Hospital. It consisted of six white tents, each with eight beds known as "cholera cots," with holes for bodily fluids to slip through. There, doctors gave him medication for pain, antibiotics to fight the disease, and salts to help his diarrhea-racked body rehydrate. They did not insert an IV, something MSF treatment centers avoided.

Khan's illness set off alarms in Freetown. Sierra Leone's national hero, a very public face of the outbreak, needed help. Government officials sent desperate e-mails to an army of experts from across the globe, in search of any kind of cure, no matter how experimental. As it happened, one possible solution, never before tried on a human, was sitting in a freezer in Kailahun.

The serum was called ZMapp, an experimental drug that had proved effective in chimps. It was made of antibodies grown in tobacco plants in Kentucky, fashioned into a compound by a small pharmaceutical company in San Diego. The three doses that made up a full treatment course were left behind by a Canadian researcher who wanted to test whether the drug could survive in the harsh tropical heat. Now, officials from the World Health Organization (WHO), the Centers for Disease Control and Prevention, Canada's Public Health Agency, USAMRIID, and MSF spent hours on the phone debating whether they could test an experimental drug—one that had never even entered the human bloodstream—on such an important patient. Garry and his colleagues, who had worked for so long alongside Khan, called everyone they could think of, demanding that Khan be given the drug. If anyone deserved it, they said, he did.

Khan was told that the debate over whether he would get the drug was happening over phone lines in Washington, Atlanta, Ottawa, and Geneva. No one asked for Khan's opinion. The Americans and Canadians argued it was worth the risk, but the decision was ultimately left to WHO and MSF. Their decision took into account the worst-case scenario: in an atmosphere in which so many Africans already distrusted Westerners in space suits, if they gave Khan the drug and he died, they could expect to confront a riot.

On July 25, three days after arriving in Kailahun, Khan was told he would not be getting the drug.

In his first three days in treatment, Khan's condition appeared stable. He moved with ease, sitting outdoors at the Kailahun clinic, speaking with visitors through a protective mesh barrier. He asked his assistant to bring a cell phone charger so he could keep in touch with friends, family, and his clinic back in Kenema.

But as the virus grew within him, Khan became weak. On the fifth day, Khan had to be helped outside; he could not sit up on his own. Another infected nurse from Kenema, arriving for treatment in Kailahun six days after Khan, found the doctor frail, but able to sit up in bed.

After medical officials decided against giving him ZMapp, Sierra Leone's Ministry of Health played its last card, desperately trying to find a

Western hospital that could treat Khan. The government hired International SOS, a French company with a jet capable of keeping a patient in isolation during flight, to evacuate Khan to another country. Miatta Kargbo, the nation's minister of health, burned up the phone lines, calling colleagues in Switzerland, the United States, Germany, and other countries: Would you take Khan, she asked, and save his life? One by one, the Western governments declined—they did not want to take a confirmed Ebola patient, and several didn't think Khan would survive the trip.

After days of haggling, one government agreed to take Khan.[11] But MSF doctors said Khan's white blood cell count was too low, making it unsafe for him to travel. By July 29, that critical count rose, though he could no longer stand on his own. Trembling with weakness brought on by near constant diarrhea, Khan asked nurses to take him outside one more time.

It was there, in the sun of the afternoon, propped on a pillow, where the hero of Kenema died. The minister of health personally called his family to deliver the news.

Khan's death hit Garry, and the colleagues who had worked alongside him for so long, hard. Somehow, perhaps to get them to back off, they had been told that Khan would get the ZMapp treatment. When he died, Garry said in an interview, his eyes growing moist, "we just assumed it didn't work." Garry learned Khan had not gotten the drug from a report in the *New York Times*.

"They lied to us," Garry said.

Sheik Umar Khan, thirty-nine years old, came home to Kenema a few days later. Five hundred people attended his solemn funeral behind the Kenema hospital where he spent his life. No others are buried near him; the only item indicating his final resting place is a slab of tiled concrete.

The new Lassa research center, funded by the U.S. Navy, bears Khan's name.

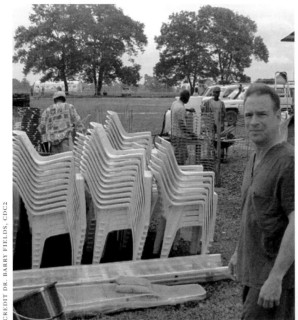

Centers for Disease Control and Prevention microbiologist Barry Fields stands outside the ELWA 3 hospital in Monrovia, Liberia. In the background, the trees under which patients waited to be admitted.

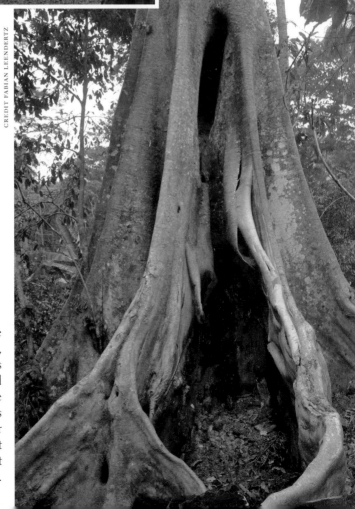

A large tree on the edge of Meliandou, Guinea, where scientists believe two-year-old Emile contracted the Ebola virus. Villagers burned the tree after the government warned against eating bush meat.

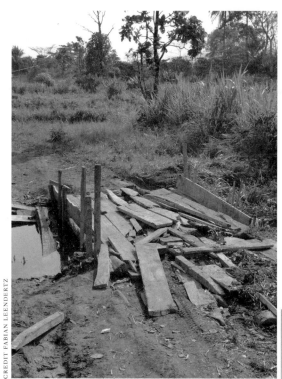

A rickety bridge stands at the entrance to Meliandou, Guinea. Neighboring villages shunned Meliandou's residents after the Ebola outbreak began.

In the streets of Meliandou, villagers hung laundry between their homes.

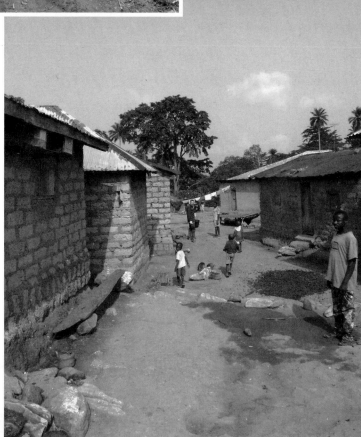

CREDIT FABIAN LEENDERTZ

CREDIT FABIAN LEENDERTZ

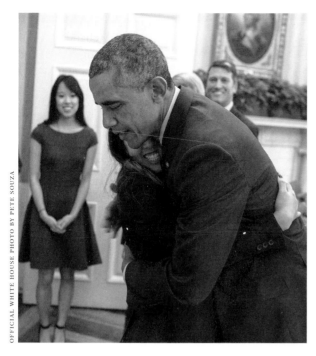

In the Oval Office, President Obama hugs Nina Pham, the 26-year-old nurse from Texas Health Presbyterian Hospital, just fifteen days after she had been diagnosed with the Ebola virus.

Obama received constant updates on the fight against Ebola. From left, Ron Klain, Ebola response coordinator, Obama, Lisa Monaco, homeland security adviser, and Denis McDonough, White House chief of staff.

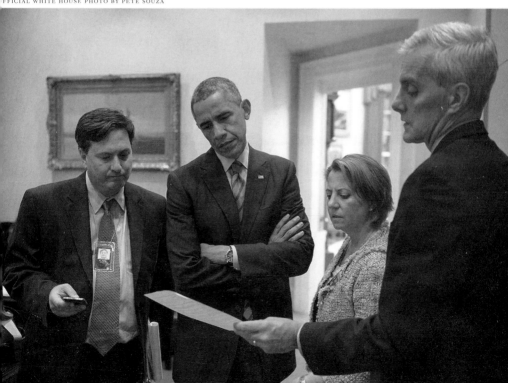

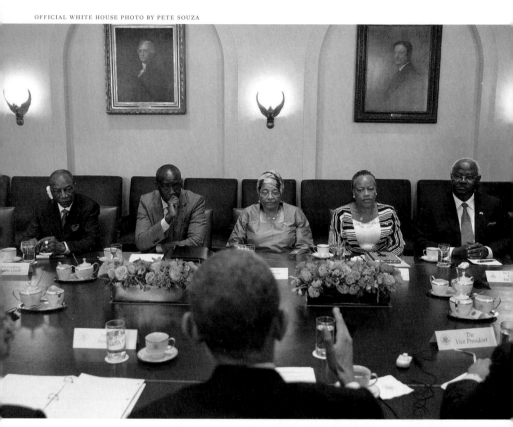

President Obama hosts West African leaders in the Cabinet Room.
Alpha Conde, president of Guinea, sits on the far left listening to the
translation; Ellen Johnson Sirleaf, president of Liberia, faces Obama; while
Ernest Bai Koroma, president of Sierra Leone, sits on the far right.

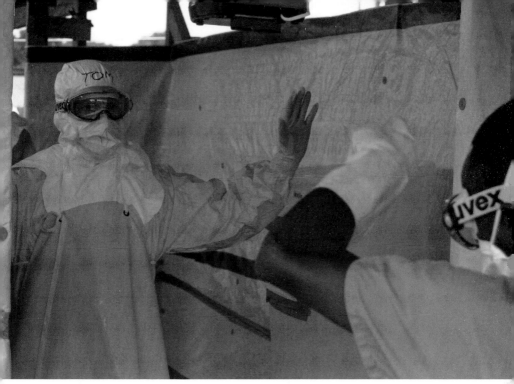

CDC director Tom Frieden undergoes
decontamination after touring the Ebola ward
at the ELWA 3 treatment unit in Monrovia.

Crosses mark the graves of Ebola victims at Disco Hill Cemetery, which
opened in December 2014. The Liberian government formally took
over management and operations of the cemetery in January 2016.

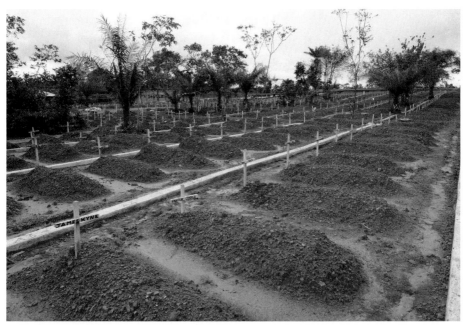

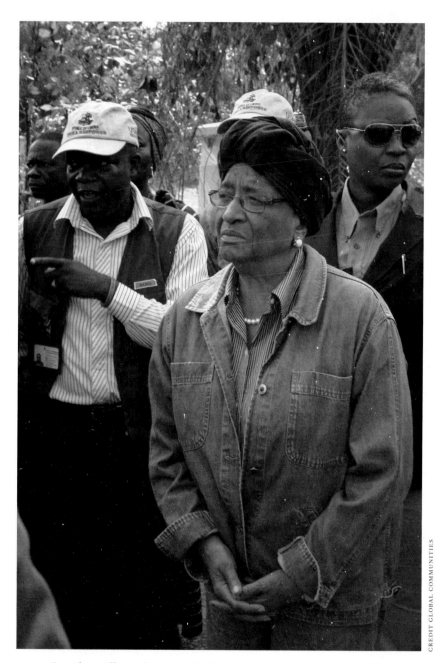

President Ellen Johnson Sirleaf tours the cemetery at Disco Hill.

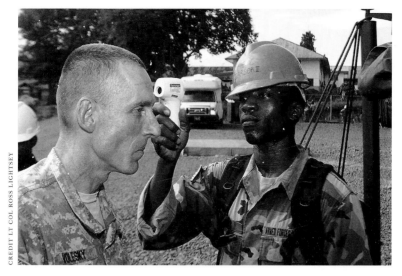

Major General Gary Volesky has his temperature taken by
a Liberian Army soldier. Although they did not come into
contact with Ebola victims, some U.S. Army officials had
their temperatures taken as often as eight times a day.

Piet de Vries, Global Communities' lead official in
Liberia, addresses a community meeting.

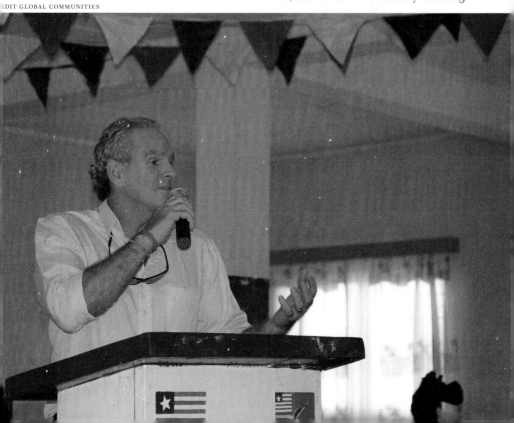

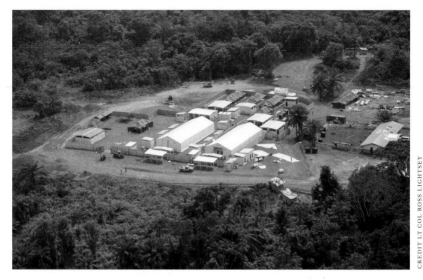

An Ebola treatment unit built by the U.S. Army, as seen from above. Patients would be treated in the white tents in the foreground. Many ETUs were built in forested areas, meaning Army engineers had to clear trees and level the ground before construction could begin.

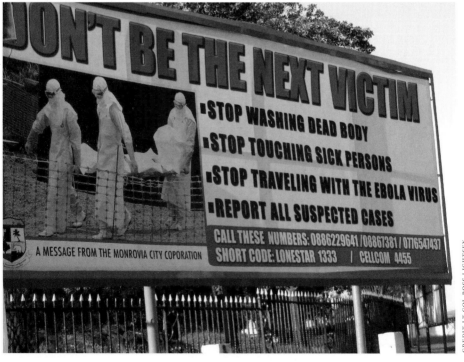

All three West African governments mounted massive public relations campaigns to raise awareness about Ebola. Here, a billboard in Monrovia warns residents to be safe around those who might have the virus.

SEVEN

Lagos

THE GLOBAL EPIDEMIOLOGY COMMUNITY is relatively small and tight-knit. Even those who see each other as rivals are cordial and close; where other academics blow disagreements over theory out of proportion, those who spend their time in the field fighting ghastly diseases cannot help but see the good in their colleagues. The death of Sheik Umar Khan, his illness apparently so mismanaged by global health authorities, enraged those who had known Khan—and, importantly, those who had been urging the World Health Organization (WHO) to stop dragging its feet and declare an emergency months earlier.

But while so many in the medical community were pulling for Khan, another potential disaster, a cataclysm that would make the outbreak in Sierra Leone, Guinea, and Liberia look tiny by comparison, was threatening about a thousand miles away. On July 20, the same day Khan felt sick enough to ask colleagues to draw his blood, Patrick Sawyer arrived in Lagos, Nigeria.

Lagos is Africa's largest city, the commercial capital of Africa's largest country. It is home to more than 20 million people, some of whom live in slums with a population density of 50,000 people per square kilometer.[1] Its population is highly mobile, both internally and externally. It is an

international city in the way Freetown, Conakry, or Monrovia are not;
Lagos's Murtala Muhammed International Airport serves international
destinations from London to Johannesburg, Istanbul to Madrid to
Nairobi—and Atlanta, New York, and Houston. Nigeria's oil and mining
industries bring international businessmen from across the globe to Lagos,
where they mingle with those who live in crowded slums. In other words,
Lagos is not only the perfect petri dish for a virus that spreads from person
to person through physical contact, it could also be the launching pad the
Ebola virus needed to go from local epidemic to global pandemic.

"The last thing anyone in the world wants to hear is the two words
'Ebola' and 'Lagos' in the same sentence," Jeffrey Hawkins, the U.S. consul
general in Nigeria, said in 2014.[2]

All Lagos needed to become Ebola's launching pad was an index case.
And to many in Monrovia's airport on the morning of July 20, Patrick Sawyer, a Liberian American lawyer scheduled to represent Liberia's Ministry
of Finance at a conference, looked suspiciously like that index case. Even
before he boarded the plane, he looked obviously ill; footage from a surveillance camera showed him lying facedown in the terminal's waiting
area. He refused to shake an immigration officer's hand, a sign he knew he
was sick. On the flight to Lagos, he vomited. He vomited again in a private
car on the way to a hospital, after Nigerian immigration officials diverted
him at the airport in Lagos. Sawyer insisted he had malaria, or something
similar; after all, he had not come into contact with any Ebola patients
back home in Liberia. Malaria is not transmitted person-to-person, so
several nurses did not bother to take precautions when checking him in.

At the hospital, however, Dr. Stella Ameyo Adadevoh suspected her
patient was lying. After twenty-one years on staff, the veteran physician
knew what she was seeing, and she knew Sawyer had something far worse
than malaria.

She was right. Weeks before he traveled, Sawyer had cared for his sister,
Princess Nyuennyue, who had arrived with her husband and her brother
at Saint Joseph's Catholic Hospital in Monrovia in early July; her husband
told doctors at Saint Joseph's that she was suffering a miscarriage. Sawyer
had paid $500 to get his sister into a private room; while the medical staff
worried the woman might have Ebola, Sawyer helped her change clothes.[3]

Princess Nyuennyue died on July 7 or 8. Sawyer, who worked as a consultant to the mining company ArcelorMittal, told his employers the next day that he had had contact with his sister. The company reported the contact to the Ministry of Health, which ordered Sawyer not to travel until he was no longer an infection risk.

Saint Joseph's itself suffered drastically. Brother Patrick Nshamdze, the hospital administrator, died August 7, buried in a mass grave that included fifty-two other victims. Seven other staff members who treated Brother Patrick also fell sick.[4] (One was Father Miguel Pajares, a seventy-five-year-old Spanish priest. He was evacuated to Spain, where he received a full course of ZMapp. The experimental drug did not work.) Weeks after its first Ebola case, Saint Joseph's, the oldest hospital in Liberia, shut down.

Before the twenty-one-day incubation period was up, Sawyer began to feel feverish. He was hospitalized on July 17, though he left the hospital, against his doctor's orders, a few days later. By July 20, he showed up at the airport for the flight, which connected in Togo, determined to deliver a lecture at the economic conference he was to attend in the Nigerian city of Calabar.[5] It is not clear why Sawyer decided to defy his travel ban. His boss at first acknowledged approving Sawyer's travel, then later reversed himself and denied issuing permission.

But while Nigeria could have provided Ebola's vault to the global stage, officials at all levels had done something those in Sierra Leone, Guinea, and Liberia had not: they had prepared. If Africa's most impoverished countries were an illustration of what happened when the global health system stumbled, Africa's most populous nation, perhaps the most potent powder keg on the continent, would become an example of what happens when the health system works as it is supposed to.

With the outbreak raging out of control a thousand miles to the west of Nigeria, the major regional hub, Nigerian health officials were keenly aware of two very strong likelihoods: first, there were enough commercial and cultural connections between Nigeria and the three West African nations that it was almost impossible to screen every traveler coming by plane, boat, or bus across their borders. Second, they knew if the Ebola virus was going to spread globally, it would likely spread by way of Lagos.

Onyebuchi Chukwu, Nigeria's minister of health, demanded his staff be ready in the event of an ill patient. Health-care workers across the country, and especially in the poorer neighborhoods of Lagos and the capital Abuja, were given crash courses in detecting a possible Ebola patient and in protecting themselves if and when that patient walked through their doors. The training was by no means comprehensive, but it was far more than health-care workers in West Africa had received.

The nation had other advantages, too: Nigeria, unlike the three West African countries that had suffered the brunt of the Ebola outbreak, has something approximating a modern health-care system. Nigeria's oil wealth makes it the richest country in Africa, and some of that wealth had gone toward building medical capacity that would now become crucial to stopping the virus before it got out of hand. The country's leading health experts also knew how to respond to outbreaks on grand scales. Though they had no experience with Ebola, Lassa was endemic to the region; that virus got its name from a small town in northeastern Nigeria, near the border with Cameroon. International organizations like the World Health Organization (WHO) and the Centers for Disease Control and Prevention (CDC) had spent decades fighting disease around Nigeria, making the Westerners in space suits known quantities both to federal and state governments and to the people they would be working to protect. Managed properly, the skepticism that international aid organizations faced in Liberia, Sierra Leone, and Guinea would not be a problem in Nigeria.

In those first hours after Sawyer landed, before most Nigerian officials realized they had their first Ebola case on their hands, they caught two crucial breaks. When Sawyer arrived on July 20, he had quickly been identified by immigration officials as a potential risk. Those officials had diverted him to a medical facility. The first break was that he had been allowed to fly at all. Had Sawyer arrived by bus, a more common mode of transportation through countries in West Africa, had he breezed by immigration agents, or had he been diverted to a public hospital, the index patient might have sparked a global catastrophe.

The second twist of good fortune appeared, on its face, as a stroke of incredibly bad luck. The day Sawyer landed, medical staffs at public hospitals were on strike. But that turned out to be a cloud with a bright silver lining: instead of being taken to one of Lagos's major medical facilities, where thousands of patients and poorly trained health workers could have been at risk, he was transported to First Consultant Hospital, a small, privately run facility led by Dr. Adadeyoh.

Three days after arriving at the private hospital, Sawyer's blood tests came back. Adadeyoh was startled, but not entirely surprised, to find that her suspicions had been correct all along: Sawyer had Ebola. The patient was less accepting of the diagnosis. Sawyer was irate. The doctors had gotten it wrong, he screamed. He insisted that he be allowed to leave. He pulled an IV line out of his own arm, spraying blood tainted with billions of Ebola virions around the room.[6]

Adadeyoh was pressured to free her patient from two other altogether more surprising sources: the Liberian Ministry of Finance and the Liberian ambassador. They both demanded that Sawyer be freed, first to continue on to the conference in Calabar, then finally, just to return home. Sawyer wanted to travel much farther than Liberia. His wife and children were waiting for him in Minnesota. Adadeyoh continued to refuse.[7]

In Abuja, news that Sawyer's blood work had come back positive set off a mad, but orderly, scramble. Chukwu's Federal Ministry of Health, CDC's Nigeria office, and the national WHO outpost, led by Dr. Rui Vaz, declared an Ebola emergency that same day the results came in. CDC director Tom Frieden, traveling in rural Kentucky and struggling to maintain a cell phone signal, tracked down Babatunde Fashola, the governor of Lagos state. "Governor, if you don't control Ebola, it's the only thing you will ever be remembered for," he warned.

Within hours, an Incident Management Center opened its doors to oversee the response. The center operated like a war room, dispatching dozens of teams to track down everyone who had come into contact with Sawyer, keeping tabs on those contacts, and mounting an aggressive public relations campaign to let Nigerians know: Ebola is here, but we are on it.

The contrast with the outbreak that began in Guinea could not have been more stark. Medical officials near Meliandou had not even suspected an outbreak had begun until two months after the toddler Emile had fallen ill. By that time, dozens had died and dozens more were infected. In Nigeria, officials knew they had their first Ebola case within seventy-two hours of his arrival.

The contrast was stark, but it wasn't entirely an even match. Nigerians had decades of experience tracking down disease—which meant the populace had years of experience with the medical system that was now mobilizing to save them. Just two years before Ebola arrived, Nigeria had stepped up its efforts to eradicate polio, which was still endemic to the region. The government had been aggressive and innovative: The program used satellite-based global positioning systems (GPS) to ensure that children living in remote villages were vaccinated.

Then, the Ministry of Health had opened an Incident Management Center to track the fight against polio. Now, many of the same people who worked in the center reprised their roles as virus hunters; the deputy manager of the center during the polio campaign was promoted to manager. The same GPS that had been used to track villages where children were vaccinated against polio were now used to keep tabs on the growing list of those who had contact with an Ebola patient, who would need to be monitored for three weeks. Nigerian health officials opened a makeshift Ebola treatment unit in just fourteen days, twice as fast as anyone else had been able to open a new facility.

The center operated as the hub from which separate spokes branched out, all working together to stamp out any chance the virus might have of escaping their ever-contracting web. Separate units oversaw the response's strategy and coordination campaigns; one was dedicated to case management, another to infection control. A media and public affairs team handled social mobilization, alerting community leaders of the virus in their midst and helping those communities build response strategies. A team of scientists oversaw any necessary laboratory services. Another team managed every point of entry into the country.

Each played a well-practiced role. The social mobilization team worked to spread as much information about Ebola as it could and to reduce the stigma of contracting the disease. (Ending the stigma, as West African officials came to learn, was critical to identifying the extent of any outbreak: if people are scared of being ostracized by their communities, they won't come forward to be treated.) They personally contacted residents in about 26,000 homes.[8] The team charged with watching ports of entry kept a vigilant eye out for anyone else who might carry the disease with them, checking temperatures of everyone who crossed into Nigeria, by plane or bus or boat. The strategy team organized shipments of protective equipment to health care centers around Lagos, then organized trainings for medical personnel.

Others worked with the media, traditional and religious leaders to teach them about the science of Ebola—the ease of transmission, the importance of getting early treatment, the danger in caring for a sick family member or preparing a body for burial following traditional guidelines. Traditional and religious leaders had worked with government officials on the polio vaccination program two years earlier. A parallel public relations campaign, broadcast over radio and television airwaves, featured prominent actors from Nollywood, Nigeria's growing and hugely popular film scene.

Most crucial were the tracers, those dispatched to find anyone who might have been infected by Sawyer. Forty epidemiologists and 150 staffers trained in the art of contact tracing fanned out across Lagos. They hunted down passengers from Sawyer's flight, the immigration officials who had stopped him, airport personnel, the driver who brought him to the hospital, any nurses or technicians or doctors who might have come into contact with him at the hospital. They searched through slums, where many of the houses had no street numbers. Any home or vehicle or public space that might have been contaminated got a thorough hosing with virus-killing chemicals.

Tracing Sawyer's contacts and the contacts of others who came down with Ebola made a massive difference. In West Africa, Ebola had spread undetected through several successive generations of victims before contact tracers arrived to identify those at risk. The aggressive contact tracing in Nigeria meant that anyone who was infected would be identified, isolated, and treated as quickly as possible, severely curtailing the number of others they might infect in turn. Second-generation spread, a key metric epidemiologists track in any outbreak, was far lower in Nigeria than it was in Sierra Leone, Guinea, or Liberia.

Even under the high-quality care of a private hospital, it was too late for Sawyer. He succumbed on July 25, just two days after his blood work came back positive. But the contact tracers were still hard at work, identifying seventy-two people with whom Sawyer had had contact between the time his plane landed and his lab results came back positive. Anyone who showed symptoms was immediately moved to an isolation ward, their blood shipped across town to new high-tech facilities at the Lagos University Teaching Hospital for testing. If Ebola was in their blood, the patient would be transferred to an equally high-tech treatment center.

In spite of the Nigerian government's quick action, Sawyer had managed to spread the disease. And as in West Africa, health-care workers once again bore the brunt of Ebola's toll. Eleven of the twenty people who would eventually fall ill in Nigeria were health-care workers. Nine of those people had contracted the disease before Sawyer's blood work came back.[9] Many did not understand how they had gotten sick.

"I never contacted his fluids. I checked his vitals, helped him with his food," nurse Obi Justina Ejelonu wrote in a post on Facebook. "I basically touched where his hands touched and that's the only contact. Not directly with his fluids." She was among the nine who got sick after treating Sawyer before his diagnosis came back.[10] So was Dr. Adadevoh. The veteran physician, the anchor of the private hospital, died August 19.

The tracers found another 279 people who had contact with others who got sick in Lagos. Just one victim managed to slip the net by flying west to Port Harcourt, Nigeria's main oil port. That patient, who left to seek medical treatment from a private physician, infected three others, including the physician, who died after two agonizing weeks, on August 23.

Again, tracers dispatched by the Incident Management Center went to work canvassing Port Harcourt. They were startled to find that the doctor had come into contact with hundreds of people in the ten days between his initial contact with his patient and his development of symptoms. Eventually, the number of contacts in Port Harcourt rose to 526—more than enough to set off an explosive outbreak in another densely populated city. Tracers kept close track of all 526 people for the three-week incubation period. Incredibly, only two got sick.[11]

By September 5, little more than a month after Sawyer's death, the last of the twenty cases of Ebola Nigeria would experience was diagnosed. Eight of the twenty patients had died, while the final patient walked out of Lagos's Ebola treatment center nineteen days later, on September 24, with a clean bill of health. On October 20, forty-two days—or two incubation periods—after the final case was confirmed, WHO officially declared Nigeria to be Ebola-free.

The spread of Ebola to one of the world's largest cities represented the worst nightmare of epidemiologists and public health officials around the globe. But while other cities might not have been ready, in Nigeria the officials had been unusually prepared to defend Lagos. The preplanning—made possible by smart investments in a solid foundation of public health and prior efforts to stamp out disease through an organized campaign—left Nigeria with a blueprint for beating back an epidemic. Every player, from the minister of health Onyebuchi Chukwu to the contact tracers walking Lagos's slums, knew exactly what they were supposed to do, and none tried to delay or deny the virus's presence. Incredibly, the contact tracers from the Ministry of Health, and another team from MSF, tracked down all but one of the 894 people who had primary contact with an Ebola victim in Nigeria.[12]

"That was the moment of maximum terror," the CDC's Frieden recalled later. "It was literally days from being out of control. [Ebola] would have been all over Lagos, all over Nigeria, all over Africa for months and years to come. This was the moment at which the world was on the brink of a catastrophe."

The city, the world, caught its share of breaks: that public hospitals were on strike limited the contacts Sawyer could have; that a sharp-eyed immigration officer spotted the ailing man. But without the years of preparation and groundwork Nigeria had laid, those bits of luck would have been but drops in the bucket. The fast action from Abuja to Lagos and Port Harcourt demonstrated how to handle an outbreak effectively enough to minimize danger, both to a crowded country and the world. They were lessons that those in Liberia, Guinea, and Sierra Leone—not to mention the World Health Organization itself—would learn from in the coming months.

EIGHT

The Samaritans

IN LATE JULY, RANDY SCHOEPP of the U.S. Army Medical Research Institute for Infectious Diseases (USAMRIID) took a rare few hours away from the diagnostics clinic he ran outside Monrovia to visit a new facility on the other side of town. It was a new Ebola treatment center, built at an existing hospital in Paynesville City, a major suburb along a bustling highway. The hospital itself had been maintained by Eternal Love Winning Africa (ELWA), a Christian missionary organization, since 1965. Now, another missionary group, Samaritan's Purse, had become the first nongovernmental organization (NGO) outside of Médecins Sans Frontières (MSF) to open an Ebola treatment center. The facility would be called ELWA 2.

Schoepp was impressed with the new treatment center. For Liberia, still struggling to build its medical capabilities, it looked relatively modern, with as many protections for doctors and nurses as one could reasonably expect in a field hospital. The unit had forty beds, making it one of the larger facilities in Liberia at the time; half were reserved for confirmed Ebola cases, the other half for suspected cases.

A bright-eyed young Samaritan's Purse doctor with closely cropped red hair named Kent Brantly guided Schoepp and a few other Army doctors around the building, showing them the new shower facilities that would decontaminate anyone walking from an isolation ward back into a clean zone. Brantly asked one of his colleagues, a Liberian nurse, to demonstrate the process of donning and doffing a protective suit; he was clearly proud, eager to show off the skill of both the American missionaries and the Liberian nurses and technicians who would staff the ward. Brantly asked what Schoepp thought, a sign of respect from one young doctor to an older, more experienced expert. Schoepp could not help being struck by his enthusiasm.

But something else struck Schoepp at the same time: Brantly didn't look terribly well. Brantly had apologized when he refused to shake Schoepp's hand when they first met, explaining he was a little under the weather. Neither the refusal nor Brantly feeling a little ill was odd. Almost no one was making physical contact amid the heightened tensions of the outbreak, and almost every Westerner making a first visit to West Africa would experience some kind of symptoms, whether a headache or an upset stomach. Schoepp thought nothing of it as he stood shoulder to shoulder with Brantly, watching the donning and doffing demonstration.

Back at the HIV diagnostics clinic a few days later, though, a new blood sample crossed Schoepp's desk. It was labeled Tamba Snell, a name he recognized, one he had seen before, and one that was obviously fake. That meant the sample probably came from an employee of a nongovernmental organization; NGOs had a habit of labeling their employees' blood samples with aliases, both to protect their privacy and to avoid the stigma of even being tested for Ebola in the first place. Schoepp thought back to the day before, when he had stood so close to Brantly, well inside the three-foot buffer zone recommended by health officials.

Then another sample crossed Schoepp's desk, another alias, Nancy Johnson. Both came back positive. He asked his sources for the real identities of Tamba Snell and Nancy Johnson. The answers: two American missionaries working at the ELWA 2 hospital. One was named Kent Brantly.

A chill went up Schoepp's spine. The fact that they stood so close together now meant that the Army doctor and the rest of his team were possible contacts, too. They spent the next three weeks testing their own temperatures at least twice a day, monitoring themselves for signs of the virus. Many times, one member of the diagnostics team would catch another with a thermometer. They exchanged knowing, fearful looks: You okay? Should I be worried? Every slight twinge or minor headache sent paranoid thoughts of Ebola racing through their heads.

Brantly was just thirty-three years old when Ebola came to Liberia. A deeply religious man, he had studied at Abilene Christian University in Texas, where he hoped to become a missionary. During his college years, he went on a mission trip providing care to poor children in Central America; it was a life-changing experience, one that convinced him that medical missionary work was the channel through which he would serve God. He earned his medical degree from Indiana University in 2009, then trained at John Peter Smith Hospital in Fort Worth, Texas, where he worked in a program for doctors who would practice in rural communities or in the developing world.

Only months after finishing his residency, Brantly, his wife Amber, and their two children had moved to Liberia, in October 2013, volunteering with Samaritan's Purse, an organization founded by the evangelist Franklin Graham. Their small home, covered by a thin tin roof, faced the Atlantic Ocean. He quickly built a reputation at the ELWA 2 facility as a man of deep compassion: When it became clear that any of the sick patients wouldn't survive, Brantly, clad in head-to-toe protective gear, would hold their hands, pray with them and sing to them.[1]

At the ELWA 2 hospital, Brantly met Nancy Writebol and her husband David, volunteers for another Christian ministry, Serving in Mission, the parent nonprofit that operated the ELWA hospital. David's job was to keep the facility running, to keep the lights on and the generators pumping. Nancy was a clinical nurse associate, given the critical tasks of ensuring that doctors and nurses were properly suited in personal protection equipment before entering the isolation wards, then spraying them down with chlorine when they came out.

It was a relatively low-risk, though crucial, assignment; a line of tape on the floor of the shower area separated Writebol, dressed in gloves and a disposable apron, from doctors and nurses in full-body suits. Writebol would also take the temperatures of family members of infected patients, though none of them showed any signs of infection.

On July 22, her fifty-ninth birthday, Nancy Writebol came down with a fever, a symptom she knew well. A few months before, Writebol had contracted malaria, and now she thought the disease had returned. She asked a Serving in Mission doctor for a malaria test, which came back positive. Writebol returned to the small home she shared with David, where she had malaria drugs in the bathroom. All she needed, she thought, was some medicine and a few days' rest.

But her symptoms kept getting worse. The fever didn't break, and soon she developed a dull, intensifying headache. On Saturday, the same doctor who had given Writebol her malaria test stopped by their house. The doctor didn't want to frighten anyone: "We're just going to do the Ebola test, to relieve everyone," she told Writebol. The doctor and David left for an all-staff meeting at the hospital, taking her blood sample with them. Writebol lay down for a nap.

A few hours later, once the samples had made their way to Schoepp's lab, Lance Plyler, Brantly's boss, got a text message from Schoepp's team: "I am very sad to inform you that Tamba Snell is positive," the message read. A short time later, Writebol's sample—labeled Nancy Johnson—came back positive, too.[2]

David returned to their house. He stood outside the door: "Nancy, I have something to tell you," he said. "Nancy, Kent has Ebola. And so do you."[3]

The doctors who had accompanied David back to his home, to give his wife such terrible news, were beside themselves. "We are so sorry, Nancy. We are so sorry," she later recalled them repeating, over and over.

Writebol was painfully aware of her odds. In the weeks since the ELWA facility had opened, she had watched forty patients enter the Ebola ward— the twenty beds for suspected cases quickly became twenty more beds for confirmed cases, and even then they had to turn potential cases away. Just one of those forty patients had survived. When the first two patients arrived on June 11, one, an older man, had not even survived the ambulance ride.[4]

In the weeks that followed, Writebol went over her time at the ELWA facility, trying to recall a moment when she might have come into contact with someone who was infected. Another technician who sprayed down doctors and nurses coming out of the isolation wards, a Liberian, had been infected a few days earlier in his community; he had come to work while showing early symptoms, but even then Writebol could not recall physically touching her colleague. She never figured out the moment at which she could have contracted the virus.

It mattered less how they were infected than how they would be treated. Plyler began making every phone call he could—to the Centers for Disease Control and Prevention (CDC), National Institutes of Health (NIH), Canada's Public Health Agency. He learned about more than a dozen possible treatments, with names like T705, rNAPc2, TKM-Ebola, and ZMapp. None had been tested on humans, though ZMapp had worked to cure monkeys infected with Ebola.

Plyler called Larry Zeitlin, the president of Mapp Pharmaceuticals, to beg for a dose. The only treatment course that was anywhere near the ELWA facility, though, was in the freezer in Kailahun, Sierra Leone, where at the same time Sheik Umar Khan lay dying. Brantly and Writebol both said they would opt for that drug, if it was available. Plyler and Zeitlin made contact with Gary Kobinger, of Canada's Public Health Agency, to try to get the drug to the nearest airstrip, across the border in Foya, Liberia.[5]

The U.S. embassy in Monrovia sent Lisa Hensley, a microbiologist at USAMRIID who had spent her career looking for possible drugs to treat hemorrhagic fevers like Ebola, to Foya by helicopter to pick up the sample. She was accompanied by a U.S. marine—just a precaution, they were told. After flying through thick fog and pelting rain, they discovered that the doses of ZMapp had already left aboard a flight chartered by Samaritan's Purse. The helo heaved back into the sky to return them to Monrovia.[6]

The three-dose course of ZMapp arrived at the ELWA 2 hospital in a Styrofoam cooler. Kobinger and others had been clear with Plyler: there is only enough medicine to treat one patient, they told him. The drug acts like a boxer fighting a particularly resolute opponent. One dose, or one punch, would knock the disease down, but it required two more punches to knock the disease out. Whatever he did, Plyler was not to split the doses between both patients.[7]

Plyler drove to Brantly's small home, where he could speak to him through the window. The young doctor was doing better than expected, hovering in stable condition. He expected to be evacuated to the United States within just a few days. Together, they decided Writebol should get the treatment. Brantly called Writebol and urged her to take the drug.

Plyler jumped back into the car, drove the short distance to Writebol's home, and handed the drug to Dr. Debbie Eisenhunt, one of ten doctors and nurses attending to the two Americans around the clock. Eisenhunt placed the first dose under Writebol's arm, where it would thaw slowly; too fast and the serum could be destabilized.

Just hours later, on July 31, Brantly began to spiral. He looked visibly worse, sweating, groaning in pain. Plyler called Brantly's wife, Amber, and Franklin Graham, to let them know. And he began to consider doing exactly what he had been told not to do—splitting the doses. Plyler unpacked the second dose and began to thaw it. Plyler closed his eyes and bowed his head: "God," he prayed, "he cannot die."

Plyler returned once again to Writebol's house, where Eisenhunt retrieved the now-thawed first dose from under Writebol's arm. They disinfected it, then wrapped it in a plastic bag, where it rode next to Plyler on the short trip back to Brantly's home. There, he handed the vial to another physician, Dr. Linda Mobula, who inserted the drug into an IV bag dripping into Brantly's arm. Plyler sat vigil outside Brantly's home as the first drops of ZMapp filtered down into Brantly's vein.[8]

Within half an hour, as the drug coursed through Brantly's bloodstream, he began to shake, a tremor at first, then uncontrollably. It was the first hint that ZMapp was having an effect. After an hour of shaking, Brantly seemed to calm. Miraculously, it seemed, his fever broke, his temperature began to return to normal and his breathing, once laborious, steadied. Even the rash on Brantly's chest seemed to fade. Doctors hooked up a new bag, this one a blood transfusion from a fourteen-year-old boy who had survived Ebola, and whose blood would carry antibodies that would give Brantly's immune system another weapon against the disease.

The following morning, Brantly stood up and walked to the bathroom. A day before, he hadn't been strong enough to stand.[9]

Writebol was not as lucky. Her first dose, the second in the course, administered beginning August 1, did not show the same instant effects it had on Brantly. In fact, she began to develop an itch on her hands, a possible sign of an allergic reaction. Her doctors dialed back the amount of serum dripping into her veins, which seemed to ease the discomfort.[10] She, too, got blood transfusions, though none with Ebola antibodies—none of the Ebola survivors matched her blood type.

Back in the United States, the White House and the State Department scrambled to find a way to get the two Americans home. They identified one company, called Phoenix Air Group, that could do the job. The company, based in Cartersville, Georgia, had a single plane that could fly a patient at Biosecurity Level 4, the most secure environment. The "air ambulance" held a sealed room behind the cockpit, which was kept at lower air pressure than the rest of the plane. This ensured that any leaks would suck air into the compartment, rather than pushing air into the cockpit.

But even with the proper equipment to transport the two patients, there were problems. The air ambulance had taken off for Liberia on July 30, the day before Brantly received his first dose of ZMapp. It had to turn back because of a pressurization problem.[11]

Finally, on the morning of August 2, Brantly walked onto the plane under his own power. It lifted off, headed back to Atlanta. After it landed at about 11:20 a.m. local time, news helicopters captured video of a man in full personal protection equipment climbing out of an ambulance and walking slowly toward the open doors of Emory University Hospital, where an isolation ward waited. He was helped by another person in full protective gear. Kent Brantly was home.

Now, it was Writebol's turn. The Phoenix air ambulance lifted off once again, bound back across the Atlantic.

But the second American was struggling. She had received two doses of the three-dose course, though she hadn't experienced the same rebound as Brantly. Doctors had trouble finding a vein to keep her IV in; they eventually put an IV directly into the bone, which caused her terrible pain.[12]

Just hours before she would take off for Atlanta, Writebol made a point of asking for her favorite Liberian dish, a potato soup. She wasn't sure she would ever have the chance to try it again; she didn't think she could survive the ten-hour flight stateside.[13] Dressed in full protection equipment, she was loaded onto a luggage conveyor belt to be placed in the level-4 biocontainment suite on the plane. One of her doctors put his hands on her mask and brought his face close: "Nancy," he told her, "we're taking you home."

On August 4, Writebol arrived at Emory too. Brantly could see her through the window of their adjoining isolation units. He tried to wave, but she was too delirious to see him.

But with constant supervision in a world-class medical facility, both patients quickly improved. A new dose of ZMapp had arrived from

Kentucky BioProcessing, the facility that made the experimental drug using tobacco plants, and both Brantly and Writebol completed their treatment courses. They discovered that small encouragements mattered. The day a doctor told her she had turned a corner, Writebol willed herself, for the first time in a week, to stand up, go to the bathroom and take a shower. Two weeks after entering Emory's hospital, Kent Brantly walked out with a clean bill of health.

The happy ending to the stories of Kent Brantly and Nancy Writebol served as a rare positive moment, and a dire warning, to the global health community. On one hand, there was now evidence that the Ebola virus could be beaten. On the other, their illnesses had virtually shut down ELWA 2, one of the only hospitals in a city of a million residents where a highly contagious disease was only beginning to spread. Three other Liberian health-care workers at ELWA 2, including Writebol's colleague, had also fallen ill. Two had died. Other NGOs saw the collapse as a particularly scary reminder of the ever-present danger. Two volunteers got sick at the first NGO other than Médecins Sans Frontières that tried to open an Ebola ward

In the United States, the sick Americans served as a catalyst for top disaster response experts, who began to realize the scale of the outbreak, and the warnings they had been hearing from Frieden, Fauci, and others.

"For us, the fact that Monrovia was now left without a net was much more concerning [than the two Americans falling ill]," said Jeremy Konyndyk, the head of the United States Agency for International Development (USAID) Office of Foreign Disaster Assistance. "From a containment of the disease perspective, what really started the alarm bells ringing was not that two Americans were sick, but that the one treatment option in Monrovia is collapsing, and there was nowhere for patients to go."

The fact that Writebol and Brantly had survived, and that Dr. Sheik Umar Khan had not, set off another debate, one that put the World Health Organization (WHO) on the spot. WHO had been cautious about using the experimental ZMapp on a human without proper trials.

"Using an experimental vaccine on human beings in the middle of an outbreak in this case would not be ethical, feasible or wise," one WHO official had told *Science Magazine*.[14] But Writebol and Brantly were alive, and Khan was dead.

On August 6, WHO changed its stance. It would convene a panel of experts to consider the ethical ramifications of an experimental vaccine or treatment.

"The recent treatment of two health workers from Samaritan's Purse with experimental medicine has raised questions about whether medicine that has never been tested and shown to be safe in people should be used in the outbreak and, given the extremely limited amount of medicine available, if it is used, who should receive it," the agency wrote.[15]

But experimental drugs are just that, experimental. And the Centers for Disease Control and Prevention wanted to temper expectations as much as they could.

"The plain fact is that we don't know whether [ZMapp] is helpful, harmful, or doesn't have any impact," CDC director Tom Frieden told a congressional committee on August 7. "And we're unlikely to know from two or a handful of patients whether it works."[16]

The message Frieden was sending was clear: The Ebola outbreak would not be stopped by a miracle drug, one that was both unproven and unlikely to be produced in mass quantities. The world needed to do more—and given that the WHO had proved so inept at accomplishing the job, the United States needed to take on a bigger role, maybe even the lead.

It was a message that would be delivered over the next month, repeatedly, as case counts mounted. By August 8, 2014, more than 1,700 total cases had been reported across Guinea, Liberia, and Sierra Leone. More than 950 people had already died. And the curve was beginning to bend upward.

NINE

A Call for Help

IN EARLY AUGUST, Liberian president Ellen Johnson Sirleaf called her chief ally on Capitol Hill, Senator Chris Coons, the chairman of the U.S. Senate Foreign Relations Subcommittee on African Affairs. Coons admired Sirleaf, a bipartisan cause célèbre in Washington at a time when there had not been many success stories in Africa. When Sirleaf was elected president in 2005 as the unity candidate capable of healing the deep wounds left over from the country's second civil war, First Lady Laura Bush and Secretary of State Condoleezza Rice had attended her inauguration. Sirleaf had given a joint address to Congress, a rare honor for a foreign leader; George W. Bush had awarded her the Presidential Medal of Freedom, the highest civilian award an American president can bestow; and Barack Obama welcomed her to the Oval Office in 2010, crediting her "heroism and courage" in helping Liberia heal. She shared the Nobel Peace Prize in 2010, an award she won for her work to promote women's rights (though the timing of that award, coming just days before Sirleaf won a second term, was not without controversy).

Coons, a freshman Democrat from Delaware, knew more about the desperate poverty of Africa than most of his colleagues. He had served as a relief worker in Kenya and written a book on South Africa during apartheid.

And he knew Sirleaf well. He had attended her second inauguration, after she won reelection with 90 percent of the vote (the opposition candidate had boycotted the election after the controversy over the Nobel Peace Prize). The two politicians, one a brightly dressed African woman in her seventies who had seen the worst of civil war, the other a low-key backbench senator with a graduate degree from Yale Divinity School, formed an unlikely bond; Coons thought Sirleaf was tough and resolute.

But now Coons heard a desperation in Sirleaf's voice. Her country, she told him, was dissolving around her, laid prostrate by a virus the public health infrastructure had no ability to defeat. The World Health Organization (WHO) was so miserably behind the curve that the number of Ebola cases was beginning to skyrocket, both in the remote rural counties up north and in crowded and impoverished Monrovia itself. Help, she said, was nowhere on the horizon.

"Everything was shutting down. They were feeling a sense of abandonment by the world. Airlines were stopping [flights], cargo ships were no longer coming," Coons recalled later. "They increasingly felt isolated."

Coons promised help. He thought he had grasped the seriousness of the situation, but when Sirleaf made a specific request for funding, Coons realized the true magnitude of the burden Liberia faced: Sirleaf's country needed help building a crematorium to dispose of dead bodies that would otherwise infect someone new. They simply did not have the space, or the time, to bury the dead.

Over the scratchy transatlantic connection, Sirleaf and Coons prayed together.

On the ground in Liberia, the situation looked even worse. In one twenty-four-hour period in the second week of August, 113 new cases were reported in Liberia alone, and the real number was probably far higher. On August 12, Mosoka Fallah, the Harvard-trained epidemiologist, found Ebola patients in West Point, the overcrowded Monrovia slum where safe sanitation was virtually nonexistent, creating an atmosphere ripe for infection. Community leaders admitted they had been burying their dead without reporting them to authorities.

"It became apparent that what we were seeing was the tip of the iceberg," Fallah recalled later. "There had been secret burials. The people had been sworn to secrecy."[1] Within weeks, victims were dying so fast their bodies were being thrown into two nearby rivers.

Johnson Sirleaf's government tried to clamp down on the outbreak in West Point, imposing a strict quarantine on the slum's tens of thousands of residents on August 19, a week after the first cases there turned up.

Most international health experts advised against cordoning off an entire Monrovia neighborhood. Doing so, they warned, would leave the impression that West Point had been left to die on its own. But Johnson Sirleaf sided with her Army chiefs, who proposed the idea in the first place.

"We have been unable to control the spread [of Ebola] due to continued denials, cultural burying practices, disregard for the advice of health workers and disrespect for the warnings by the government," Johnson Sirleaf said in a statement announcing the quarantine the night before it took effect, issued after most West Point residents had gone to bed for the evening. "It has thus become necessary to impose additional sanctions."[2]

The riot police and Coast Guard units who showed up the next morning to enforce the quarantine met crowds of angry West Point residents. Groups of young men threw rocks and attacked riot police, who showed up one Wednesday morning to enforce the lines of demarcation. Thousands of residents worried they would not be able to get to their jobs in other parts of the city. A fifteen year-old boy, Shakie Kamara, died after being shot in the leg during the clashes. More people might have died had not a torrential rain storm sent people fleeing back to their homes.[3]

Many residents disregarded the quarantine on a regular basis. Some swam around the quarantine lines. Others slipped through loosely-guarded sections. There was no shortage of soldiers willing to accept a few dollars in bribes in exchange for turning a blind eye to the escapees.

Those who left were more worried about starving to death than about contracting Ebola. Thousands lined up every day, waiting in lines for government handouts of rice and water as a thriving black market for other goods flourished.

Johnson Sirleaf toured West Point a few days later, surrounded by heavily armed guards in protective gloves who kept the angry crowd away from Liberia's president at what may have been her government's lowest ebb during the outbreak. She apologized to Shakie Kamara's family for his death. Though she did not make any public comments during her visit, a man in her entourage threw wads of bills at some of the loudest protesters— quieting their yelling, but sparking fist fights over the cash.[4]

Days after the president's visit, her government lifted the quarantine. It had not done much good, even as a public education campaign.

"Most people here still don't believe there is Ebola in West Point," the manager of a drug dispensary told a reporter for the *New York Times*. "They're saying that the government came and didn't find Ebola, and so that's why they're leaving."[5]

The disease was decimating more than the bodies of the victims themselves. Pillars of society—a very vulnerable society at that—began to shut down. Businesses closed. Food and fuel were in short supply. Regular health services, in a region where malaria was a constant danger and where the infant mortality rate was among the highest in the world, collapsed almost entirely. Because caring for a family member who is ill or the body of one who has died falls to women in West African society, a huge number of pregnant women were becoming infected. Rick Brennan, head of WHO's emergency assessment team, called delivering a baby in Liberia "one of the most dangerous jobs in the world."[6]

Nongovernmental organizations (NGOs), whose selfless labor was desperately needed to stem the spread of Ebola, were looking to the U.S. embassy for guidance. The embassy had held a town-hall meeting for NGOs in late July to review safety protocols, to reassure nervous ex-pats that contracting Ebola wasn't likely if those safety protocols were observed, and to send the clear message that embassy personnel were not leaving.

On July 30, the Peace Corps said it would pull its combined 340 volunteers out of Guinea, Liberia, and Sierra Leone. After half a century in existence, the Peace Corps had developed a reputation as one of the last organizations to leave a dangerous situation; their exit now spooked the NGO community, which had already been shaken when Brantly and Writebol fell ill. Many organizations made their way to the airports as fast as they could. Others were forced to leave when their insurance providers hiked premiums through the roof.

As those groups departed, the United States Agency for International Development (USAID) Office of Foreign Disaster Assistance (OFDA) was considering ways to join the fight. But it was not clear that an agency more accustomed to fighting famine or providing relief from a devastating hurricane or earthquake would be able to add anything to a fight against a disease that the Centers for Disease Control and Prevention (CDC), or the WHO, or Médecins Sans Frontières (MSF), were not already doing.

The American in charge of the OFDA was Jeremy Konyndyk, a tall and lanky thirty-six-year-old who had worked in refugee camps in Guinea during the Liberian civil war. In early July, he had dispatched Justin Pendarvis, a USAID public health adviser with years of his own experience in West Africa under his belt, to evaluate the situation on the ground. In the space of just a few weeks, Pendarvis observed Ebola treatment units in Conakry, Guinea; Kenema, Sierra Leone; and Monrovia, meeting with teams from the CDC, MSF, WHO, and the United Nations to see what USAID might add. USAID, after all, was full of disaster response experts, not outbreak response experts; historically, the two communities of specialists had viewed each other with suspicion.

Pendarvis bridged the gap between the two communities, and his years in West Africa gave him more insight into what he was seeing. Yes, he concluded, USAID needed to get on the ground—and fast.

Not every NGO had pulled out, and counterintuitively, the absence of so many groups made coordination among those that remained more efficient. In an ordinary disaster response, representatives from perhaps dozens of NGOs will crowd into a massive conference room or community center in an attempt to coordinate efforts; groups shouting over each other is not uncommon, according to those who have been involved in previous disaster relief efforts. In the three West African countries, in late July and early August, the coordination meetings could happen around a single table at a local café, or in a government minister's small conference room.

Pendarvis had already identified the few groups that were left. The Liberian Ministry of Health's main organizational group, the Incident Management System, would be chaired by Tolbert Nyenswah—a lawyer by training with a master's degree in public health from Johns Hopkins University—who served as the nation's assistant minister of health. When it was established, Nyenswah's group was focused on Monrovia, where Ebola had the potential to explode within crowded slums. But to get a better handle on what was happening in the northern counties, where the disease had first crossed the border from Guinea, Pendarvis turned to Global Communities and its in-country director, Piet deVries.

DeVries had spent about a decade traveling back and forth from his home outside Washington, D.C., and Liberia, where Global Communities was running a USAID–funded program called Improved Water, Sanitation and Hygiene, IWASH for short. As part of that program, Global Communities had created a network of emergency health technicians (EHTs)—if there is one group that tends toward confusing acronyms more than the U.S. government, it is the community of nongovernmental organizations— who worked in the rural northern counties.

Those EHTs, always local Liberians, had spent years going to small villages working to create a mental link between the proximity of latrines and a water source and corresponding incidences of cholera. They were technically employees of the Liberian Ministry of Health—U.S. federal law prohibits paying foreign government employees a salary—and now they were beginning to use their connections with local villagers to establish burial teams, which they hoped would cut the chain of transmission by safely laying to rest anyone who had died of Ebola.

DeVries told Pendarvis that his EHTs were receiving the equivalent of just US$80 a month, and getting only minimal training from the Liberian Ministry of Health and the WHO, for performing one of the most dangerous jobs around. Lofa County, where the first burial teams were built, had offered an additional $20 per burial for each member of the team, but the county government soon ran out of money. DeVries asked USAID for money to pay the burial team member bonuses. The wire transfer took place in a matter of days. Soon, USAID sent Global Communities more money to pay for new burial teams in Bong and Nimba Counties, two more northern outposts where Ebola was burning fiercely.

DeVries used some of the money to supply his EHTs himself; materials the burial teams needed to do their jobs safely were arriving in Monrovia by the boatload, but they languished in warehouses, waiting for shipments north, which never took place. One hot morning in mid-August, deVries picked up 5,000 body bags at a warehouse in Monrovia and drove them north to Lofa. When deVries arrived, he found the first burial teams wrapping bodies into plastic sheeting, because they had run out of body bags of their own.

In Washington, officials had begun meeting to figure out how they could assist. Gayle Smith, the senior National Security Council (NSC) staffer with a long background in Africa, began convening meetings of what is known as an Interagency Policy Committee, a group of top-ranking representatives from relevant agencies, on July 22. She began holding daily meetings of NSC staff tasked with scaling up international efforts the following week, on July 28. Three days later, on July 31—the day Brantly received his first dose of ZMapp—the White House held its first principals-level meeting, which included national security adviser Susan Rice, Samantha Power, the American ambassador to the United Nations, and health experts like Tom Frieden of the CDC and Anthony Fauci of the National Institute for Allergy and Infectious Diseases (NIAID).

Those early meetings focused on the most basic elements of an outbreak response—how to build an Ebola treatment unit, how to usher a patient from a waiting room to a diagnostics area and, eventually, to an isolation ward. Rajiv Shah, USAID's administrator, had his staff put together PowerPoint slides that showed the floor plan of a treatment facility. Jimmy Kolker, the assistant secretary of Health and Human Services for Global Affairs, offered to deploy a team of doctors from the U.S. Public Health Service's Commissioned Corps, an agency that ordinarily sends medical professionals to impoverished communities around the United States. Fauci routinely briefed the president himself, beginning in early August, when Obama asked for an outline of the science of Ebola.

On the sidelines, Frieden and Fauci, who ordinarily chatted several times a week about whatever was happening in the global health world, were talking daily. So too were Shah and Sylvia Matthews Burwell, the secretary of Health and Human Services. Fauci was routinely on the phone with Lisa Monaco, the White House's top homeland security official, and with Denis McDonough, President Obama's chief of staff. Shah spent hours on the phone with Sirleaf and her two counterparts, Guinea's president Alpha Conde and Sierra Leone's president Ernest Bai Koroma, fielding requests for aid and receiving updates on the extent of the outbreak.

The sense among senior American officials, from the White House to the CDC and National Institutes of Health (NIH), was that the Ebola virus still represented a threat almost exclusively to the three West African nations, and not to the United States. The difference between public health systems in Liberia and America was equivalent to the difference between riding a bicycle and traveling by jumbo jet; few top officials seriously worried that the virus would make its way back to American shores. That gave the White House the sense that they did not need to overcommunicate, in the words of one senior administration official. They didn't need to sound alarms about a threat they saw as remote—a decision several said in hindsight they would regret.

There were some early signs that the American public saw the threat of an outbreak on American soil as far more likely than the White House did. On August 1, 2014, less than a year before he would kick off his improbable presidential campaign, Donald Trump tweeted to his millions of followers: "The U.S. cannot allow EBOLA infected people back. People that go to far away places to help out are great-but must suffer the consequences!" Nearly 4,300 people retweeted Trump. A subsequent analysis by the White House Office of Digital Strategy found that Trump's tweet had captured Americans' worries about the virus. "It was that tweet that created a level of anxiety in the country," Amy Pope, a senior White House counterterrorism official, said in an interview. "That was a crystallizing moment."

Unbeknownst to Trump, he had tweeted at exactly the moment when some officials at the National Security Council and the State Department were worried for the first time that Ebola could hop a plane across the Atlantic. The occasion was the African Leaders Summit, which brought heads of state from fifty African nations to the Mandarin Oriental Hotel, the State Department headquarters, and the White House. The summit would focus on trade and investment between the United States and Africa; commerce secretary Penny Pritzker announced nearly a billion dollars in new international deals during the three days when motorcades shuttled senior officials across a gridlocked capital. Guinea's president Alpha Conde, Liberia's vice president Joseph Boakai, and Sierra Leone's foreign minister Samura Kamara, all attended with their retinues. Johnson Sirleaf and Ernest Bai Koroma, Sierra Leone's president, stayed home.

Pope worried that the summit, which included dozens of staff, hangers-on and members of the African media attached to each delegation, might inadvertently serve as the opportunity for Ebola to spread, either between delegations or to civilians in the Washington area. Homeland Security officials and the CDC trained the Secret Service, who would be deployed to protect and watch visiting African dignitaries, to spot signs of Ebola. High-level meetings were held to decide whether someone who exhibited a cough should be let in to official events. Pope breathed a sigh of relief as the African leaders left on August 6, after none had shown obvious signs of being sick.

Meanwhile, the National Security Council sped up its plans to dispatch aid back across the Atlantic. At a meeting of top NSC deputies on August 3, the White House agreed to Shah's recommendation that they send a formal USAID team—known as a Disaster Assistance Response Team, or DART—to Liberia. The following day, Deborah Malac, the American ambassador in Monrovia, formally declared a disaster, paving the way for a DART deployment.

The first DART team on the ground in West Africa arrived in Monrovia on August 7. Shah and Konyndyk at USAID, Smith at the White House, Fauci at the NIH, and Frieden at the CDC had already concluded that the WHO was in over its head, with central leadership in Geneva badly disconnected from the grim reality on the ground. They were shocked, nonetheless, that it took WHO until August 8 to declare the outbreak a "public health emergency of international concern," its highest threat level. The declaration came almost four and a half months after the first Ebola case was announced, four months after MSF had declared an emergency, four days after the U.S. ambassador had issued her own formal warning, and a day after the first significant U.S. presence had already landed.

Sending in DART represented a major escalation of American involvement. The team included representatives from the Department of Defense, the Department of Health and Human Services, USAID, and CDC. It consisted of logisticians who would help deliver crucial supplies to Ebola treatment units, burial teams, aid workers, and anyone else who needed help; disaster response experts who embedded within Liberia's Ministry of Health to support Tolbert Nyenswah, heading the emergency response at the Incident Management System; communications specialists, who fought with Liberia's unreliable telecommunications systems to make sure the team had a reliable line to Washington and Atlanta; a safety and security officer, who did everything from protecting team members on their travels to and from work to speaking with staff at the team's hotel, to ensure that proper hygiene techniques were being followed; and even a medical officer, who would constantly check on team members themselves, to make sure no one was coming down with anything—whether malaria or Ebola.

The team, ordinarily sent to the site of a disaster response rather than a viral outbreak, was meant to pave the way for future American investment and to ease the strain on an embassy in an affected country. One embassy is not equipped to handle or coordinate a full-on disaster response; DART parachutes in for the ultimate in crisis management.

USAID, rather than sending thousands of its own responders, instead typically identifies and funds other groups, like Global Communities and Samaritan's Purse, that execute relief efforts on the ground itself. Still, the dearth of NGOs meant that these DART members had to act quickly, on their own. Early on, a group of team members fanned out across Monrovia, scouring markets and shopping centers for every ounce of chlorine they could find, and spray bottles too. They packaged those supplies up by hand and sent them to every Ebola treatment unit they identified around the country.

The remaining NGOs started seeing money from American coffers in short order. USAID had already started funneling money to some organizations; in March, it had sent $600,000 to the United Nations Children's Fund (UNICEF), which was working on rapid response. By the time of DART's arrival, the spigots of American dollars were opening, from a trickle to a gusher. Within two days of showing up, the team had approved $14.6 million in USAID funding, on top of $2 million already sent to WHO. Three days later, USAID said it would send another $7.5 million to Liberia, which would pay for 105,000 sets of personal protection equipment. Another three days later, a second team was deployed, this time to Sierra Leone.

At the same time that the DART members arrived, and while burial teams began operating in northern rural counties, the Liberian government was having trouble finding space to bury bodies in Monrovia. About 70 percent of all Ebola transmissions came from contact with dead bodies, which became festering cesspools of virus; finding a safe way to remove those bodies was essential, outbreak specialists knew, to ending the chains of transmission.

But early efforts to create a safe burial space ran into local roadblocks. When the Ministry of Health tried to bury thirty bodies at a site near Monrovia, they had to call in security officers to fend off nearby communities that did not want a cemetery in their backyards. Once the residents were gone, an excavator plowed a mass grave. But the ministry had picked a low-lying area at the peak of the rainy season. As the water table rose, it brought bodies floating back up to the surface. It was a major embarrassment for Sirleaf's government, which was already straining to prove it could handle the crisis.

The Ministry of Health hit upon a new solution, one Sirleaf brought up to Coons in that early August phone call: they needed to burn the bodies to kill the virus.

But cremation is a foreign concept to most Liberians, for whom the ritual of preparing a body for the afterlife was an important cultural touchstone. The thought of burning bodies was unpopular with many Christian Liberians, and even more so with the significant Muslim population.

"The idea of burning bodies is unpalatable in Liberia," deVries explained. "It doesn't happen."

It was so unusual that Liberia did not even have a crematorium capable of handling the bodies. Instead, they borrowed a facility owned by the Indian Embassy; for Hindus, cremation is a cultural tradition. On August 5, the Liberian government ordered every corpse in Monrovia to be burned.

Even then, the government proved to be unprepared, thanks in large part to woefully inadequate record-keeping. A major part of Liberian funerary tradition revolves around having a place to mourn the dead. At government-run Ebola treatment units in the city, however, ashes were put in barrels, with no record of whose remains were lumped together. Families that had worried about relatives going into an Ebola treatment unit and emerging as corpses now worried that they wouldn't even have a corpse to bury and mourn. Patients who died at facilities run by Médecins Sans Frontières could count on excellent record-keeping, but it was cold comfort for those whose relatives died lonely, painful, frightening deaths.

The cremations also fed a growing sense that some victims of the Ebola virus were being treated differently than others, exacerbating tensions that had lingered since the nation's devastating civil war between the governing elites—the descendants of freed American slaves—and the tribes that had lived in Liberia for millennia. Many governing elites continued to bury their dead, even though government policy explicitly called for cremations.

At one meeting of a committee dedicated to dead body management, held in a Ministry of Health conference room and attended by senior officials from MSF, Global Communities, the CDC, and the WHO, the woman who chaired the meeting told the shocked crowd of humanitarian responders she had just come from a funeral herself. The Liberian official in charge of enforcing cremations was violating the rule she was meant to enforce.

Zanzan Kawa, head of the Traditional Council of Chiefs and the highest-ranking tribal leader in Liberia, had tacitly accepted the need for cremations, but he sent a powerful message when he saw the different ways his people and governing elites were being treated: They're not burning the elites, he said. They're burning us.

The NGO community was unanimous in warning the Liberian government about the danger it was courting: You're creating a disconnect between the elites and the poor, they told the government. That disconnect threatened to undermine the careful relationship that NGOs were building with the very poor, those who stood the highest risk of catching Ebola because of their close-quartered living conditions and lack of available hygiene. Without that foundation of trust, the NGOs warned, more people would go into hiding rather than seeking treatment, exacerbating the spread of the deadly disease.

On August 17, about two and a half weeks after the ELWA 2 hospital had collapsed under the weight of the two sick Americans, MSF once again stepped in to fill the breach. It opened a massive new clinic in Monrovia called ELWA 3—at 120 beds the largest Ebola management center ever built. Still, the facility was not big enough, and MSF doctors had to turn away clearly sick Liberians simply because there were no beds to hold

them. Those who were sent away were given home protection kits to reduce the risk of infecting their families at home.

"The numbers of patients we are seeing is unlike anything we've seen
in previous outbreaks," an overwhelmed Lindis Hurum, MSF's emergency
coordinator in Monrovia, said just a few days later. "Our guidelines were
written for an Ebola center with 20 beds, and now we are expanding beyond 120 beds."[7]

Like its predecessors, the ELWA 3 facility did not resemble a Western
hospital. Instead of brick and mortar, patients rested under a series of tents,
donated by various government and nongovernment agencies. Fences made
of rebar and door flaps separated red zones, where Ebola patients were
quarantined, from safe zones, presumably free of the virus. Patients waiting to be admitted lounged under two tall trees outside the hospital; responders called them the Ebola trees.

Barry Fields arrived at the hospital a few days before it opened. Fields, a
microbiologist by training, had been based at CDC's Kenya office for
three years. A few days after Kevin De Cock, head of CDC's Kenya office,
left to head up the agency's response in Liberia, he called Fields and told
him to pack his things. Liberia needed more diagnostic capability, and
Fields had the equipment necessary to rapidly build up a laboratory for
testing blood samples of potentially infected patients.

Initially, Fields and his colleague Heinz Feldmann, chief of an NIH
virology lab at the Rocky Mountain Laboratories in tiny Hamilton, Montana,
planned to set up their operation in Lofa County, in the rural north. But
when they arrived in Monrovia in August, another senior CDC official, Joel
Montgomery, told them the plans had changed. The virus was erupting in
the slums of Monrovia, and they were needed in the capital.

"We need to control this thing here," Montgomery told Fields. "It's
going to explode in the city."

The lab equipment Fields packed up included seven hundred pounds
of gear, including generators to keep the delicate and highly technical machines whirring. With it, he could build a level-3 biosafety lab in the field,
capable of protecting scientists and technicians from the worst bugs on
Earth. But the contractor they had recruited to ferry the gear to Liberia

had trouble with the customs paperwork, holding up their mission for three long days.

In the interim, Fields met with staff from Médecins Sans Frontières, to plan where exactly they would set up the lab. The MSF staff had been laboring to get more than a few blood samples tested each day. When Fields told them how many samples his machines could process—about 150 a day—their jaws hit the floor. On the spot, they volunteered to give Fields and his team as many construction workers as they needed. Once construction began, the rudimentary laboratory was completed within twenty-four hours.

Still, the lab was primitive at best. Like the ELWA hospital itself, Fields's team operated in an open-air tent, stocked with plastic patio furniture they had purchased at a local hardware store. The August monsoons beat down on the roof constantly, and they had to hire a Liberian man to sweep out the rain. They worried constantly about being electrocuted, or that the water would short out their pricey gear. They bought fans, too, in a perpetually losing battle against the tropical heat.

Once the customs paperwork had been fixed and the tent erected, the complicated system of testing blood samples took on a regular order: Fields or one of his colleagues would collect samples from a refrigerator just outside the red zone, walk past patients waiting to be admitted under the Ebola trees, and place the blood in an acrylic box. The blood would be treated with a buffer solution that extracted RNA, which would prove whether Ebola was present in the blood, while killing 99.9 percent of the virus. They added an ethanol solution to kill what virions remained, turning the blood a rust brown color.

The treated samples would then be moved to two extraction machines, which would amplify a few pieces of RNA so that the computers could tell whether a sample had Ebola present. The two machines were able to diagnose a sample with near-perfect accuracy; to be certain, they ran each sample through both machines. Results were entered into a computer, which would then be sent to the appropriate hospitals.

The tent was situated along the main walking path between the road and the ELWA hospital. As patients walked down the path, they frequently stopped by the lab tent in search of treatment. Fields and his colleagues had to direct them to the hospital itself, though they could tell how sick many were.

"You just knew they were dead," Fields said later, mist coming to his eyes.

In its first week of operation, the CDC team scanned three hundred samples, a huge improvement over the seemingly interminable waits doctors and patients had to endure before. But the results were as depressingly monotonous as the rain that beat on the roof: Positive. Positive. Positive.

The results were so grim that they had to find solace in any way they could. When the first survivor walked out of ELWA under his own power, having beaten Ebola, Fields, Feldmann, and their colleagues snapped photos with the healed man.

But more patients arrived seemingly by the hour. Taxis carrying the sick would pull up to the ELWA hospital, where a team would help the patient inside while another team sprayed the vehicles down with a chlorine solution to kill whatever virus particles remained behind.

Each day was a brutal slog. A Liberian driver would pick them up at their beachside resort, the same hotel where Randy Schoepp and his team were staying, at 8:00 a.m. They spent most of the day testing samples from patients at ELWA, subsisting on Pringles and cookies for lunch. As the sun set, invariably new samples would arrive from John F. Kennedy Hospital on the other side of town. Well after nightfall, they drove back to the hotel. They took what little pleasure they could in a friendly competition with the U.S. Army Medical Research Institute for Infectious Diseases team, comparing how many samples they had each tested that day. They rarely mentioned how many had come back positive.

Exhaustion set in, and nerves increased. When Fields scraped his arm on some rebar, where patients regularly rested, his colleagues tried to reassure him that he wasn't at risk, that almost certainly any virus particles that remained had died after being exposed to the air and sun. Fields seethed. "It isn't your damn arm," he thought.

A few days after a Western doctor stopped by to see their facility, a sample with the doctor's name on it came through their lab—and tested positive. The team spent days replaying their meeting in their heads: had they shaken his hand? Every few minutes, it seemed, one of them sneaked off to take his or her own temperature to check for symptoms. (The doctor, whose name was never disclosed, was evacuated to the University of Nebraska, where he was nursed back to health.)

Bleach was everywhere. The person who collected samples from the hospital fridge would bleach his or her hands and boots on the way in, and on the way out. Fields wears a sterling silver wedding band; by the time he returned home, the band was black from constant bleaching.

The ever-present fear of the Ebola virus played out at home, too. A photograph of Fields appeared on the front page of USA *Today*, above a story about another Western health-care provider who had been exposed. The implication that Fields was the one exposed sent his family into a frenzy, before he could assure them he was okay.

The ELWA hospital struggled to accommodate the demand from patients infected with Ebola. Within ten days of the facility's opening, MSF technicians were already working to build three new tents, each capable of housing another 40 beds. Ultimately, the facility grew to a capacity of 250 beds; during the course of the outbreak, it treated 1,909 patients, 1,241 of whom tested positive for Ebola. Of those cases, just 541 survived.

The flood of American aid continued through August: On the twenty-fourth, USAID airlifted more than 16 tons of medical and emergency equipment to Monrovia from a forward-staging warehouse in Dubai. The shipment included another 10,000 sets of personal protection equipment, two water treatment systems, two portable water tankers, and 100 rolls of plastic sheeting to construct new Ebola wards. Three days later, Shah authorized another $5 million from USAID's coffers.

The next day, August 28, 2014, a new WHO count showed a total of 3,052 confirmed Ebola cases in the three West African countries. Liberia had reported a jump of almost 300 cases in just a week. Already, half—1,546 souls—had died.

Sirleaf's call for help, along with increasingly urgent on-the-ground reports from Pendarvis and others, had spurred a flood of relief from an increasingly attentive American government. But there was little evidence that the early efforts were working; the case count was spiking upward at a faster rate than even the most pessimistic projections. It was fast becoming clear that a more aggressive response was essential to bending that curve downward. What was less clear was just how anyone—the American government or the global health community—could provide that more aggressive response.

T E N

70–30

AFTER A MONTH OF increasingly alarming reports, Jeremy Konyndyk decided he needed to get a firsthand sense of the scale of the outbreak, and Tom Frieden decided it was time to create a more formal structure to respond to the outbreaks. International panic was growing; between the time Konyndyk and Frieden booked their tickets on a British Airways flight through London's Heathrow Airport, and the day the flight left, the airline had canceled its routes to the three West African nations. Konyndyk and Frieden had to scramble to rebook a Delta flight to Ghana, and to connect from there to Monrovia (British Airways was not alone; of 590 monthly flights to Guinea, Liberia, and Sierra Leone, 216 had been canceled by mid-August, an airline data provider reported).[1]

When they finally landed, the two Americans were immediately struck by the deeply worried mood they encountered. At one of their first meetings, with Ellen Johnson Sirleaf and her advisers, Konyndyk was struck by how grim the room seemed. Everyone was scared, and everyone was exhausted. They showed him a chart illustrating the virus's explosive growth in recent weeks, a line that grew exponentially into a mountain of disease and death. There had been more cases reported in a single day earlier that month than during the totality of most previous outbreaks.

Frieden had arrived with the goal of organizing the chaotic response. None of the three West African countries had tapped a single person to oversee the governments and nongovernmental organizations (NGOs) now rushing in to help, and no one seemed to be taking the basic steps necessary to provide the number of beds necessary to quarantine patients, provide them with care, and stop the virus.

"You hit the tipping point when the Ebola treatment units [ETUs] got full. And that was for a few reasons," Frieden said later. "One, they got unsafe, and health care workers got infected. Two, people couldn't come there, so they went back to the communities and spread [Ebola] widely. Three, the care in the ETUs was so poor at that point that people said, Why go there? It's just a place to die."

In July, Frieden had thought they would need to build facilities capable of housing three hundred patients—one hundred in each country—to stop the virus. But that meant building other infrastructure as well. They would have to organize staff to care for the patients, transportation for those who might be sick, and laboratories to sample blood. It was an enormous logistical undertaking, unlike any even the Centers for Disease Control and Prevention (CDC) had attempted in years past. And as each day passed, the number of beds they would need to control the spread of the virus increased.

"The painful fact was, we knew in July if we could get 300 beds, we could end it. By November, we needed 3,000 beds," he recalled later.

Frieden delivered a blunt message to Sirleaf: The world will not come to your aid fast enough. It was not possible for the world to marshal assistance fast enough. You have to mobilize your own communities, spread as much information as possible, while the disjointed international response got its act together.

The first task was to organize a single point person to run the entire response. In Liberia, that person was Tolbert Nyenswah, head of the Incident Management System. The IMS had become the common means by which the CDC handled outbreak responses, and increasingly the way other humanitarian groups organized responses, in the wake of the September 11 terror attacks in the United States. The goal, Frieden explained, was to take what seemed like a dauntingly massive problem—an international outbreak of a deadly virus—and break it down into solvable problems. "Instead of having a fog of war experience with just chaos going on, it's a way of structuring your emergency response," he said. "If you have a big problem, break it down to less big problems, and then solve each of those less big problems individually."

Nyenswah chaired the daily meetings, which took place in a huge conference room in central Monrovia. Government agencies, foreign governments, nongovernmental organizations were all present, and teams tasked with tackling every aspect of the response would deliver daily status updates. Every meeting was heavily structured, to waste as little time as possible. Precision and timeliness were critical: briefing memos laying out decisions ahead had to be delivered on time, and once a decision was made, tasks needed to be tracked. Final decisions rested with Nyenswah, the unflappable deputy minister of health with an education from Johns Hopkins in Baltimore. Everyone else scaffolded, in Frieden's words, around him. Ordinarily, someone who will run an IMS undergoes months of training. Nyenswah dove in with little more than a briefing from Frieden and his team.

While in Monrovia, Frieden and Konyndyk visited the huge ELWA 3 facility, run by Médecins Sans Frontières (MSF). Konyndyk was horrified to see patients being turned away. Just weeks after opening, the Ebola treatment unit was already full. Frieden was equally horrified to see the conditions inside the treatment center, where 125 patients were being overseen by a single doctor, Armand Sprecher. Sixty corpses lay scattered about the makeshift hospital, some lying dead right next to patients still struggling for their lives. Diarrhea, blood, excrement were everywhere. The nurses and technicians left alive to tend to the hot zone could not clean up fast enough. It was, Frieden recalled, like something out of Dante's Inferno.

Konyndyk himself had seen the aftereffects of Liberia's civil war, and the long road to recovery the nation had walked; this was worse. "They're a very resilient country. They're no strangers to tragedy and crisis," he recalled later. "But this was just totally unfamiliar."

It became clear that the situation was unfamiliar to the NGOs on the ground, too. Konyndyk and Frieden came away from a meeting with World Health Organization (WHO) officials deeply unimpressed by what they heard. Konyndyk and Frieden were "absolutely on fire," Konyndyk said later. "We were being outpaced by the disease. We were losing."

After Konyndyk returned to Washington, Frieden continued traveling through Guinea and Sierra Leone, where he told their presidents what he had told Sirleaf. He was struck by the differences in each country's approach: Sierra Leone was employing its military far more than the other two nations, and imposing curfews on villages and communities where the virus was present, sowing even more distrust between traditional villages and the central government.

In Guinea, President Alpha Conde had implemented a practice his government called micro-cerclage: The military and police would arrive in an infected village and surround it, though residents were still free to come and go. Anyone leaving simply had to leave their cell phone number with guards, so they could be tracked. The government shipped in food and medical supplies, so that a village did not get the sense that it was being shut off from the outside world and left to die.

"We have an expression in the U.S.: You catch more flies with honey than with vinegar," Frieden told Conte.

"Yes," Conte replied. "But the honey has to get there before the flies leave." Frieden was struck by Conte's underlying point: his government was building trust. Breaking the vicious cycle of mistrust between government and community, Conde believed, would break the virus's back.

Konyndyk was still contemplating how his office, the Office of Foreign Disaster Assistance (OFDA), could best contribute to the effort. He and Frieden both concluded America needed to ratchet up its response, and quickly, by building new Ebola treatment facilities and sending hundreds, maybe thousands, of medical personnel. But OFDA was not equipped to handle a response of the magnitude necessary. Even the CDC wasn't technically in the disaster response business. Konyndyk and Frieden started to throw around ideas of just who could handle such a mammoth response. They settled on one outside-the-box possibility, the only agency that could marshal thousands of people with cutthroat efficiency: the United States military.

Back home, the American response was taking shape: the United States Agency for International Development (USAID), through OFDA, led the effort, coordinating and managing logistics and procurement. The CDC was the deputy lead, with primary responsibility for the science and epidemiological elements.

The Americans had a model, one that suggested how to bend the curve downward. Based on previous outbreaks, the virus would eventually be contained if they could isolate 70 percent of those infected—completely isolate 30 percent of all infected patients in Ebola treatment units, and partially isolate another 40 percent, at home and away from family. Even if the remaining 30 percent were not isolated, statistical analysis suggested that they would not be able to infect enough friends, family, and neighbors to keep the disease spreading. Trying to isolate everyone, given the scary growth curve and the number of contacts each of those patients would have had, was not practical. "Once you had a massive urban outbreak, at this scale and pace, you're not going to isolate all those people," said Raj Shah, Konyndyk's boss at USAID.

Under this strategy, eventually, the virus would run out of fuel. Inside the CDC, and eventually at the White House, the strategy became known as 70–30, for the percentage of patients partially or totally isolated and the percentage responders could afford to miss. But even reaching 30 percent completely contained was a threshold of staggering proportions: by August, just 18 percent of patients with Ebola were being cared for in hospitals.[2]

In the White House, President Obama was keeping close tabs on the virus's spread, a topic now being covered daily in his early morning security briefings. Several times, he made calls to members of USAID's Disaster Assistance Response Team (DART), calls that boosted morale in Monrovia.

Obama also made calls to foreign heads of state, working around the United Nations and the WHO to solicit commitments of support. He asked for health-care workers, construction material, and manpower to build new Ebola treatment units and, critically, logistical help in ensuring that the international community had the ability to evacuate any aid worker who might get sick in the course of treating patients. Many nongovernmental organizations had communicated to Shah, Konyndyk, and others that the prime concern keeping them out of the fight was the worry that they wouldn't be able to get one of their own out of the country if the worst happened.

For weeks, Gayle Smith would make the walk across the small driveway separating the White House from her office in the Old Executive Office Building. She sat in the Oval Office as Obama contacted presidents and prime ministers from across the globe. Canada, historically reluctant to get involved in foreign engagements, especially outside its sphere of influence, declined to make serious commitments beyond its public health service. Governments in South Korea, Japan, and Germany gave freely of their money and manpower. In early October, Obama called Stefan Lofven, who had been installed as Sweden's new prime minister just days earlier. Congratulations on winning election, Obama told him. Now send money to West Africa.

Obama also spoke with China's president, Xi Jinping, about sending help. The administration had spent years carefully courting Xi and his predecessor, coaxing China onto the world stage. China's growing influence and its desire to become a world superpower were leading to investments in foreign nations, including in Africa, where it could mine precious resources for its booming manufacturing industry. Foreign policy experts in the United States, conscious that they could not contain China but eager to manage its emergence on the world stage, tried to convey to China's leaders there was more to being a superpower than just extending tentacles to other corners of the world for industrial purposes; with power comes responsibility, including the responsibility to respond in humanitarian crises.

Smith repeatedly cornered the Chinese ambassador to Washington, hammering a single message: the United States and China, she told him, were the only two countries big enough to sit on the infection curve and bend it downward. The ambassador took note; he later told a State Department official, weighing his words carefully, that Smith "is very passionate."

The Chinese were intrigued. The CDC had worked in conjunction with its Chinese equivalent, the Chinese Center for Disease Control and Prevention, since the 1980s on health crises that would occasionally pop up in Asia. Now, the Chinese agency agreed to send doctors and technicians to West Africa to help respond. They peppered the CDC in Atlanta with technical questions about how to build an Ebola treatment unit, and how to protect its citizens in the hot zone.

The African Union, eager to show its own ability to contribute to a crisis in its own backyard, sent hundreds of doctors to the scene, seeded by money from the United States, the European Union, and China.

At the same time, the coordination between the U.S. Army Medical Research Institute for Infectious Diseases (USAMRIID) and the Food and Drug Administration (FDA) were paying off. The chemical compounds Army scientists had sent to the FDA for pretesting, a deal negotiated by David Norwood, began deploying to West Africa, to speed up the diagnosis process and reduce the time between a patient's first contact with medical professionals and confirmation that Ebola was or was not present.

Norwood began shipping new assays, the chemicals that would create a visible reaction if Ebola virions were present, both to Liberia and to public health department labs in all fifty states, in the event that Ebola ever reached American shores. It was the first significant step a federal government agency had taken to reassure American governors—many of whom were getting nervous about the prospects of an Ebola outbreak in their backyards—and the public. But Norwood's decision also sent an important message to the Liberian government, where some were skeptical that their populace would be used as test cases for unproven vaccines and medicines: The very same assays that would test American blood, Norwood made clear, would test Liberian blood. There would be no double standard.

Along with the new diagnostics tests, USAMRIID deployed teams of physicians and technicians to every American hospital where Ebola might show up, to evaluate plans for isolation wards and safety precautions. Eventually, about fifty hospitals were certified to handle patients with viral hemorrhagic fever.

USAMRIID was also starting to hear from pharmaceutical companies, both big and small, that had experimental compounds that might aid in the fight against Ebola. The economic calculations necessary to invest in a treatment for Ebola were complicated. It costs millions of dollars to develop a new drug. And while a treatment for something common like high cholesterol would allow a company to recoup those research and development costs many times over, a treatment for something as rare as Ebola would not pay similar dividends. Even if a company charged hundreds of dollars for a course of treatment, earlier outbreaks had been so small that the company would only be able to sell a few hundred doses a year, at most.

Testing any potential drugs was made almost impossible, too, because none of the pharmaceutical companies experimenting with new compounds had access to a disease like Ebola. It is easy to find a laboratory rat with high cholesterol, but the government isn't about to allow a private company, no matter how trustworthy, to possess viral hemorrhagic fevers outside of the tightly controlled, highly secure labs at Fort Detrick or in Atlanta.

But other factors led pharmaceutical companies to send compounds to be tested. For a small firm, developing a landmark treatment for something like Ebola would lend a level of prestige that no amount of money could buy. For larger firms, which were slower to send their own prototype drugs, providing an answer to Ebola was less about breakout prestige or financial gain and more about demonstrating their philanthropic work.

All told, some sixty-two compounds—some potential vaccines, others potential cures—made their way to USAMRIID laboratories, where Army scientists led by Dr. Travis Warren ran exhaustive batteries of tests. Each compound was tested for toxicity, to make sure a drug would not kill a patient before it killed the virus. Then they were tested in vitro on human cell lines infected with Ebola. If those tests went well, rodents and primates were next. At each stage, scientists would measure the antiviral activity of a compound against the Ebola virions.

Even if results looked promising, there could be hurdles in production and manufacturing. One reason so few doses of ZMapp were available was that the companies that developed the drug had only limited abilities to produce the compounds from which it was made. While testing took place, the USAMRIID scientists would try to learn from the companies that created each compound whether they had the ability to produce it in mass quantities. The best drug in the world, after all, isn't any good if it can't be manufactured with sufficient speed.

By the first week of September, as the Disaster Assistance Response Teams found their footing on the ground in Liberia and Sierra Leone, as Konyndyk and Frieden contemplated how to ratchet up the American response, as President Obama worked the phones, and Army scientists ran every test they could think of, USAID's DART members in Monrovia got their first major infusion of new help. On September 9, about 100 medical professionals, including 25 doctors and 45 nurses, arrived. That moment offered a window into the speed at which the United States had ramped up its response: By then, just a month after DART had landed, USAID money was already funding 1,000 Ebola treatment unit beds.

At the same time, the WHO was starting to explore new ways to engage critical communities, to inspire some badly needed trust. Beginning in September, WHO technicians began traveling from village to village in hard-hit Lofa County, in northern Liberia, just across the border from the outbreak's epicenter. They began challenging chiefs and religious leaders to take more of their own responsibility for fighting a disease that was killing their people. The communities created their own task forces to spread word that the disease was real. To dispel ugly rumors about what happened inside an Ebola treatment unit, newer facilities would include see-through windows in the plastic walls, so that families would be able to lay eyes on a loved one.

Across the border in Sierra Leone, the country's president decided to impose a mandatory three-day lockdown, beginning September 19. Some health officials were worried that such a harsh government action would undermine the already-tenuous trust they needed to build with the community to find new cases. Others said it would allow health workers to find patients more effectively, by going house to house.

Yet while the American public was only now waking up to the tragic crisis unfolding in West Africa, two news-making moments were about to catapult the outbreak above the fold in every major newspaper in the country.

The first came on September 11, in the pages of the *New York Times*. In an op-ed piece, Michael Osterholm, the director of the Center for Infectious Disease Research and Policy at the University of Minnesota suggested there was something scientists had been afraid to say: that Ebola could mutate and become airborne.

"You can now get Ebola only through direct contact with bodily fluids. But viruses like Ebola are notoriously sloppy in replicating, meaning the virus entering one person may be genetically different from the virus entering the next," Osterholm wrote. "If certain mutations occurred, it would mean that just breathing would put one at risk of contracting Ebola. Infections could spread quickly to every part of the globe, as the H1N1 influenza virus did in 2009, after its birth in Mexico."[3]

The op-ed caused a minor panic at the White House, and at the National Institutes of Health (NIH). On Pennsylvania Avenue, President Obama's top advisers were cognizant of the politics—especially with an election just around the corner in November. They had worked hard to portray an administration capable of handling an outbreak, a government competent enough to protect its citizens. Hinting at the notion that Ebola could become airborne, which is exactly what happened in the 1995 movie *Outbreak*, loosely based on Richard Preston's book, also suggested that Ebola was destined to spiral out of control.

At the NIH, the panic bordered on apoplectic rage at Osterholm. He had given voice to a doomsday scenario, one seemingly so unlikely from a scientific perspective that even talking about it as a possibility could do more harm than good.

Obama summoned Tony Fauci to the White House for an explanation. Ushered into the Oval Office, Fauci saw that Obama was not amused.

"Tony, explain to me what that's all about," the president said. "Could it go airborne?"

In his dealings with President Obama, from the H1N1 outbreak to the H5N1 virus and other moments of public health crisis, Fauci had come to appreciate Obama's interest in and understanding of scientific rationality. Other Obama aides describe the president as a geek, someone fascinated by the intricacies of the latest research. Fauci appealed to Obama's inner scientist, though his own training demanded he hedge at least a little bit.

"In biology, you never say never, and you never say always," Fauci began. "It isn't impossible. But the chances of that happening are so vanishingly small that it's beyond a distraction. We have more important things to worry about."

"Why are you so reasonably sure about that?" Obama wanted to know.

Fauci explained the structure of the Ebola virion, what science knows about its ability to survive and thrive when exposed to various conditions. Ebola cannot survive in the air; it needs a liquid substance in which to live, like blood or other bodily fluids. The notion that a virus that has existed in that form, presumably for thousands or millions of years, would suddenly become airborne, Fauci explained, was almost inconceivable. The difference between what Ebola was today and what it would take to become airborne was an evolutionary chasm that was just too wide to fathom.

"If you look at the history of virology, viruses have mutated, a lot, always. Sometimes they become a little bit more virulent, sometimes they become a little less virulent, sometimes they get a little bit more efficient," Fauci told the president. "But there are no instances that we know of, in the history of virology, where a virus has completely changed the modality of how it is transmitted."

But Fauci recognized that a pivotal line had been crossed in the American consciousness. While scientists can be rational—and while even presidents in times of crisis are capable of logical thinking—the human brain is conditioned to react to new threats in far different ways than it reacts to old, more common threats. Humans fear being struck by lightning or being attacked by a great white shark far more than they fear being struck by a car. Statistically, that is a completely illogical construct: thousands of Americans are struck and killed by cars every year; a bad year for shark attacks might mean half a dozen victims. We fear any new terror, no matter how improbable the odds, much more than those we have been warned to avoid since we were children.

"Just because something is a new risk," Fauci explained later, "doesn't mean it's a greater risk than everything else in your life."

Obama understood the point: the op-ed would sell newspapers, and it would give Americans something new to fear, but it did not represent the realistic thinking of the scientists he was relying on to reverse the outbreak.

The second news-making moment that sent Ebola responders reeling came not from an outside source, but from within the government itself. On September 23, data analysts at the Centers for Disease Control and Prevention released a new modeling tool to project just how bad the Ebola outbreak could become. The analysis, led by noted modeler Martin Meltzer, combined every factor it could, assuming—reasonably, to most of those responding to the crisis—that reports from the World Health Organization had significantly understated the number of Ebola cases in the three West African nations, by a factor of two and a half. They offered a careful assessment of the situation on the ground, the need to isolate as many patients as possible, and efforts already being made by USAID, the Departments of Defense and Health and Human Services, and global partners to ramp up the number of available treatment beds.

But reporters covering the story, and the editors who needed a strong headline to drive reader interest, skipped over much of that to focus on a single, shocking number—the CDC's model suggested that if nothing was done to control its spread, as many as 1.4 million people could be infected by the Ebola virus by January 20, just four months down the road. That top line number was shocking: it meant the population equivalent to San Antonio, Texas, America's seventh-largest city, could be infected with one of the most deadly and horrifying diseases ever encountered by man.

In the days leading up to the CDC's stunning projections, the harmonious working relationships among the country's top health officials started to fray. The CDC had included as many caveats as it could. The projections assumed a high number of unreported cases that had yet to be discovered. The 1.4 million number was an absolute worst-case scenario that no one expected to reach, a figure that represented the natural spread of the virus if no one bothered to do anything to fight it.

But Fauci knew that reporters would only focus on that worst-case scenario. He called Frieden, the CDC director, to complain. So did USAID's Rajiv Shah and Health and Human Services scretary Sylvia Matthews Burwell. Together with the White House, they begged Frieden to present a more measured assessment that factored in all the work that had already been done to stem the virus. The numbers were flawed, they all argued, because the outbreak didn't exist in a vacuum. The ambitious response already begun by the United States, its international partners, and the three infected countries themselves were the opposite of a vacuum.

The outraged calls were not only coming from Washington. Margaret Chan, director-general of WHO, called, followed by the presidents of Liberia, Guinea, and Sierra Leone. At a time when the few global responders who were on the ground in West Africa were desperately trying to attract new help, both from other governments and from NGOs that had stayed on the sidelines out of fear, such an extreme projection would only hurt their ability to attract new aid and investment.

"That number was complete horseshit, and everybody knew it from the beginning," one senior public health official who called Frieden to complain said later. "It was nuts. It was absolutely inaccurate the minute it came out."

Frieden, unbowed, stood by his analyst Meltzer. The two men had stayed up late into the night for several days before the model was released, reviewing again and again the factors that went into the assessment, and the number that came out. The CDC has always been independent of Washington politics—part of the reason it is headquartered hundreds of miles away, in Atlanta—and Frieden was determined to protect his analysts from what might be viewed as interference. Privately, Frieden was "pissed," he later said, at the pressure he was receiving.

"We've got to tell it like it is," he said. "We have to mobilize a response and we have to be very specific about what's needed. That model was very specific: Fix the burial teams first, and second, get safe care."

Frieden took no small amount of satisfaction when, months later, the CDC's projection of what would happen if the response were ramped up mirrored almost exactly the actual number of cases and deaths on the ground. Forget the media's hyperventilating about the top line number; the analysis had been correct.

Even before the CDC's terrifying new numbers came out, the most ambitious assault on Ebola had begun to take shape. The assault had its roots in the conversations Konyndyk and Frieden had begun even before their journey through Liberia, where an idea had been born that percolated to the highest levels of the National Security Agency. It would come to a head on September 11, 2014—three days after the WHO reported that 4,269 West Africans had become infected. Of those, 2,288 were dead.

ELEVEN

Darkest Days

THE CENTERS FOR DISEASE CONTROL AND PREVENTION (CDC) sit on a pristine campus in the Druid Hills neighborhood of Atlanta, on land donated by Emory University. Gleaming modern buildings have been erected in recent years to replace older facilities, and the perfectly land-scaped grounds, populated by groups of serious-minded experts having lunch outdoors or strolling between offices can make the place feel like the headquarters of a Silicon Valley tech giant.

On the third floor of the CDC's main tower, however, the Emergency Operations Center (EOC) has a more urgent feeling. On a normal day, the several hundred computers, arranged in rows facing large display monitors that show everything from CNN to computer-generated maps and graphics, the EOC monitors everything from outbreaks across the world to flare-ups of some disease as routine as the flu back in the United States. The people who occupy those desks represent different divisions within the CDC—logistics, personnel, transportation, epidemiology, and others. Other desks are reserved for liaisons from partner agencies, the military, or nongovernmental organizations (NGOs). Bordering the room on the right side is a row of emergency operators who oversee any ongoing or emerging disasters. In the back, senior officials can be briefed in a conference room that looks over the entire EOC.

By the close of summer, virtually every desk in the EOC was dedicated to some aspect of the response to the Ebola virus. Communicating across divisions of an agency that can sometimes be too insular was critical: When Tom Frieden or the EOC manager on duty led briefings in the crowded conference room, every word spoken was broadcast into the EOC itself, and every slide the agency's leaders saw was displayed on the monitors in the main room, so no one was kept out of the loop.

The urgency that thrummed through the operations center reflected a larger state of change within the CDC. Since its founding in 1946, the CDC had routinely dispatched its experts to global disease hotspots, whether it was combating polio, malaria, Ebola, or any of a hundred other deadly bugs. But the scale of the teams that would fly out of Atlanta's Hartsfield-Jackson International Airport was relatively small. The agency had a habit of patting itself on the back when they got fifteen epidemiologists out into the field. To respond to the Ebola outbreak, especially as the case curve grew at an alarming rate, the CDC would need to dispatch a hundred times that number.

And the case curve was shooting skyward: in the first week of September, responders had identified almost 900 new Ebola victims, the number of cases had jumped from 3,052 on August 28 to 3,944 on September 6. Ten days later, another thousand people had been infected. A week after that, the case count was up to 5,843. As of September 22, 1,008 Guineans had contracted Ebola. Sierra Leone was dealing with 1,813 cases. And an incredible 3,022 Liberians were sick with the disease. The major outbreak in Lofa County had spread south and east to Bong and Nimba Counties, while another viral epicenter in Monrovia spread into Montserrado and Margibi Counties, along the coast.

But as the situation grew more grim, the CDC began its remarkable evolution. Hundreds of epidemiologists, virologists, lab technicians, and rank-and-file doctors volunteered to deploy to West Africa to lend their assistance. Some would become contact tracers. Others would monitor ports and borders. Still others would trek through the dense forest and canoe up remote rivers to advise far-flung villages on quarantines and other preventative measures. French-speakers were the most valued. Anyone with even a rudimentary memory of their high school French classes would be sent to Guinea, where the outbreak was showing new life. In all, 1,897 CDC staffers would deploy to Liberia, Guinea, and Sierra Leone in the subsequent months.

Those staffers felt a sense of duty, but also a sense of excitement. Here was their opportunity, they knew, to exercise their very specific skills to bring to heel the biggest public health crisis in a generation—maybe of their whole careers. For half a century, CDC legends had been sent to fight the most deadly outbreaks the world had ever known, and now a new generation would have the chance to add their names to the history books. They were not excited by the outbreak of a virus, they were excited about the chance to kill the virus.

But when Leisha Nolen landed in Freetown in early August, the region she had visited only a few months earlier demonstrated just how much work she and her colleagues had ahead of them.

Nolen, a thirty-seven-year-old Harvard-trained pediatrician, was one of a few dozen members of the CDC's Epidemic Intelligence Service,[1] a postgraduate course that prepares the next generation of virus hunters. She had been among the first to travel to Liberia in mid-April, first to Foya in northern Lofa County, just across the border from the outbreak's epicenter in Guinea. After three weeks, she drove south to Monrovia. At the time, no new cases popped up in Liberia, and Nolen flew home, hopeful that the disease had exhausted itself.

But even without any new cases, Nolen spotted something that concerned her: funerary traditions required Liberians to wash their dead before burial. That would put the family of an Ebola victim in close proximity to the virus at a time when the body was most infectious. The international health community could warn Liberians all they wanted about the dangers of funerary traditions, but Nolen worried that the pleas would fall on deaf ears. Those traditions were deeply woven into Liberian society, she saw, and no one gives up their cultural traditions easily.

In August when Nolen deployed for the second time, this time to Sierra Leone, she found a situation very different from the one she had left in April. In Freetown, the Ministry of Health was scrambling to respond. Few NGOs were operating at a high level. There were just two working ambulances in the entire country, and the beginning of the rainy season meant that many of the already-difficult roads became impassible. The system, Nolen recalled later, was "completely overwhelmed."

Nolen and her team of six other CDC workers soon grew to fifteen. They spent their days tracking down trucks that could be used as ambulances, dispatching body management teams and identifying new clusters of Ebola. Some of the decisions the team was asked to make were moral dilemmas with no clear answer: One day, a colleague called Nolen looking for an ambulance to take an infant showing symptoms to an Ebola treatment unit. They couldn't find a car seat for the child, and putting the baby in someone's arms for the six-hour drive to the hospital would mean putting that person at risk. Eventually, they decided to strap the baby into a basket and hope for the best. The infant made it to the hospital, but it did not survive the disease.

Through August, September, and October, almost every story ended the same way: Liberians, Guineans, Sierra Leoneans, and their international partners went to extreme lengths to get their neighbors, friends, and families to treatment centers, and those people almost always died. The growing case counts wore on doctors and health-care workers who succumbed, in their darkest moments, to fears that they were hopelessly behind the curve.

"Most of us who were there had a really hard time imagining how we were going to stop it," Nolen said later. Nolen returned from her second deployment in a state of near depression. Normally physically active on a regular basis, for three weeks, she did nothing but sit on the couch.

As the case counts mounted, the CDC dispatched more and more experts to West Africa. Peter Kilmarx arrived in Freetown, Sierra Leone, in mid-September, to lead the CDC's response from there. His plane landed after midnight, and he did not make it to his hotel until 6:45 a.m., less than an hour before his first meeting of the day. Kilmarx's team headquartered themselves at the Radisson Blu hotel, where the thirty-person team met in a boardroom with about a dozen chairs. As the team grew, Kilmarx moved the daily status meetings to the hotel restaurant, then to a three-hundred-seat ballroom they called the Cave.

Day after day, the reports were the same: supplies were limited, infections were showing up in new villages, and the response was clearly falling short. If he was lucky, Kilmarx would manage four hours of fitful sleep a night.

As CDC staffers poured in to West Africa, Kilmarx and his colleagues made sure they followed four strict rules meant to keep them safe. They were never to enter an Ebola treatment unit, a hot zone off limits to all but those directly responsible for patient care. They were never to provide direct patient care. They were not allowed to collect specimens, which needed to be handled by specially trained researchers following highest bio-security protocols. And they were never to interview a possible Ebola contact from within three feet.

The CDC grappled with the way it would treat returning Ebola workers. Ultimately, senior officials decided against a mandatory quarantine once a health-care worker returned to the United States—but doctors and investigators returning from West Africa would have to call in to both a CDC operator and the health department in their home state twice a day for three weeks, to keep an eye on their temperature.

The physical distance required to keep them safe, paradoxically, was another source of stress for many of the responders. Joe Woodring, the CDC doctor who deployed twice to Liberia and Sierra Leone, recalled the strain of staying away: "I am used to playing with kids on the street, holding the hand of a patient or giving big hugs to my CDC colleagues," he told a conference in September 2015, nearly a year after his first deployment. "This disease was too virulent and transmissible" for any of that.

Woodring reached Monrovia for the first time in mid-October. He spent his first several days squirming through seemingly interminable meetings at the embassy, antsy to get out the door and begin practicing the craft for which he had trained his entire professional life. Finally, he asked the deputy director to send him to the rural north, to the heart of the outbreak.

The CDC sent him to Nimba County, where he found two standoffish World Health Organization (WHO) officials skeptical of his arrival. Why, they wanted to know, was the CDC showing up just now?

The CDC's mission spanned from the immediate needs of dead body management to the long-term goals of encouraging behavior change among at-risk communities. It had to help ferry supplies and samples over treacherous roads, too. Back in Monrovia, laboratories worked to link strains of the disease together, to paint an accurate picture of how Ebola had spread, and to extrapolate how it would spread in the future. In Atlanta, others studied what procedures had worked and, as importantly, what was not working, to alter their tactics and strategies accordingly.

Hundreds of experts like Woodring were there to convey guidance from national health officials to the local level. The physicians on the ground in the rural north still needed basic training in practical skills, such as how to properly mix chlorine solution to wash their hands and how to don and doff the protective gear that would keep them safe. Nimba County alone had about sixty-five outpatient facilities, where an Ebola sufferer might first encounter the health infrastructure. Each one, dotted along bumpy, rutted dirt roads with mud pits half the height of a vehicle, had physicians, nurses, even receptionists who needed training.

In Nimba, Woodring awoke every morning in a virtually empty hotel once occupied by migrant workers plying the nearby mines. When the outbreak hit, the migrant workers had vanished. But the hotel's owner, a relatively wealthy man in an impoverished region, had stayed open. Woodring asked him why. Every one of his employees, the man said, was supporting seven to ten relatives. Without the wages he paid them, those dependents would starve. He stayed open to give his employees a chance to feed their families.

Fear was palpable in the northern counties. Residents were so afraid of Ebola that many were genuinely relieved to discover they were infected with malaria—a disease that kills half a million people a year. Woodring spent his Saturdays in a small town called Saclepea, where a college student, now without classes to attend, had started a new radio show to spread information about Ebola. Woodring and other CDC doctors spent hours taking calls from local villages, giving advice on how to prevent the disease from infecting new people.

On the weekdays, Woodring bounced along tracks that could barely be called roads, traveling from village to village in a special Ebola response ambulance, a modified Toyota Land Cruiser. Along one road, the vehicle became stuck in a mud pit so deep they couldn't even open the car doors. Amara, their driver, climbed out the window, hooked the Land Cruiser up to a bulldozer and pulled them free.

Along the way, as he delivered CDC flyers showing how Ebola was transmitted and how to prevent its spread, Woodring was stunned by the heroics he saw among the facilities he visited. In one village, four physicians and fifteen nurses at an outpatient eye clinic had transformed their single building into an Ebola treatment unit, without being asked, without being paid.

At another training session, at a small but surprisingly advanced facility deep in the bush, Woodring briefed the handful of health-care workers who would come into contact with any Ebola patients. The facility was one of the better medical outposts in Nimba County, about the length of a tractor trailer, painted light blue. There was no brick, but wooden walls separated different rooms, one of which served as a birthing suite. Construction of a new wing was under way, though the outbreak had halted work. Still, the local doctors had the drugs necessary to treat malaria or cholera, both of which frequently haunted their little village. The building even had a small lecture hall, where Woodring set up his presentation.

He had come armed with a mishmash of slides from the international organizations fighting Ebola. Some carried the CDC logo. Others were donated by Médecins Sans Frontières (MSF) or WHO. One slide, from the Liberian Ministry of Health, showed precautionary steps that health-care workers had to take, in excruciating—and, to Woodring, painfully obvious—detail. One step that seemed laughably clear: Change gloves between each patient.

"It's really important that you switch up the gloves," Woodring told the group as he clicked through the slides. One physician, sitting in the back, broke out into a broad smile, a grin that unnerved the American. "I'm curious to know what's funny about what I just said," Woodring told the man.

"You talk about changing gloves between patients," the physician answered. "We have no gloves to wear."

Two weeks before his arrival, the tiny Ebola treatment unit had taken in three confirmed Ebola patients. Without gloves to treat them safely, the doctors had used the only thing within reach to shield their hands: plastic bread bags. The taxi driver who had brought one of the patients protected himself by turning his jacket inside out. A shiver went up Woodring's spine.

The lack of basic medical supplies had plagued the rural regions of all three countries for months. The supply, in fact, did exist: nongovernmental organizations had shipped gloves and aprons and body bags and spacesuits into Monrovia and Freetown and Conakry by the planeload, and warehouses in all three capitals groaned under the weight of lifesaving materials. But those supplies were not being distributed to the field, where they were most desperately needed.

In some more remote areas, Ebola victims had trouble even getting to a treatment facility. David Blackley, another Epidemic Intelligence Service officer, was dispatched to Bong Town, a settlement that began in the 1950s as a home for miners who excavated iron ore at the nearby mine. There, local health officials were using an old soccer stadium as a quarantine site for those who might have come into contact with Ebola. The United Nations Children's Fund had donated four large tents, which gave health officials a rudimentary way to segregate the sick from those who did not show symptoms. Still, the families who arrived had to sweat out the equatorial heat with little hope of finding shade. Similar stadiums in small towns across the rural north served similar purposes, and local officials and their international partners cycled through a series of names for these facilities—Ebola care centers, community care centers, holding centers. Their very existence highlighted the fact that there weren't enough beds to treat Ebola patients.

The situation in Bong County also illustrated the difficulties of logistics in a third world country. When Kim Lindblade arrived from the CDC in October, she found that the official in charge of disease surveillance did not even have his own vehicle. When he could borrow one, the man didn't always have the petrol necessary to get it moving.

Blackley and Scott Laney, another CDC epidemiologist, began traveling through northern Liberia, touching base with public health officials in other remote rural regions as part of a CDC plan known as the Rapid Isolation and Treatment of Ebola (RITE) strategy. They crashed in whatever local guesthouses and small hotels they could find as they dove ever deeper into the bush. But accommodations were at times scarce. After being dropped off by a U.S. military Black Hawk helicopter in a remote part of Gbarpolu County, the team slept on the floor of the local church, after they moved the pews out of the way.

At every turn, they were attended by Isaac Kamboe, a young Liberian man of about thirty who told them about his small family. Kamboe began as the team's driver, navigating the tricky and treacherous roads. Soon he became a much more integral player, translating the local Bassa dialect into English, making connections with local tribal leaders where the Americans could not, and helping track down potential victims who had fled into the bush in fear. Within a few weeks, Blackley and Laney were including Kamboe in their daily planning and strategy meetings. His opinions had become as valuable as those of other team members who had gone through years of formal training.

Almost every team the CDC sent into Liberia had an Isaac Kamboe, a driver whose knowledge of local customs would be invaluable to outsiders. And many of the drivers had long histories of working with Americans. After the Peace Corps pulled out of Liberia, drivers who were once employed shuttling volunteers from place to place signed on with the CDC, swapping pay stubs from one American agency for another.

At times, the West Africans working alongside CDC colleagues served as chilling and important reminders of what was at stake. On another deployment, Leisha Nolen watched as the young Sierra Leonean woman assigned to enter case data found her own aunt's name in the roster of new patients. Over the next excruciating days, on the papers she handled the woman watched her aunt's life come to a slow end. She updated the case file as the older woman was admitted to an Ebola treatment unit, as her condition deteriorated, and when she died.

By the early fall, as case counts continued to rise, the early skepticism about Ebola had almost entirely vanished from rural, remote villages. Traditional leaders more openly engaged with outsiders, be they Americans or health officials from the central government, which they still distrusted. But enforcing quarantines for a family of an infected patient could, and did, lead to heated tempers and shouting matches. Few CDC officials felt as if they were in any real danger, though occasionally their local minders had to step between them and someone who might have had too much to drink.

But those in the field knew danger was ever present, and that a single wrong move could put dozens of people at risk.

Dan Martin saw the Ebola outbreak as a test of his own personal values. A pacifist, he felt called to serve something greater than himself, but he could not bring himself to sign up for the military. Instead, deploying to West Africa was his chance to make a big difference in the world. Soon after he landed in Freetown, he and John Redd drove north to Makeni, the fourth-largest city in Sierra Leone, which lies near the border between Bombali District and Tonkolili District. Martin would be in charge of the CDC response in Tonkolili—Tonk, in local shorthand—while Redd managed Bombali. They swapped notes every night by the pool at the Wusum Hotel, over dinner and a few local Star beers.

Redd was struck by efforts the hotel's proprietor made to maintain a sense of normalcy. One night, when he dropped his laundry off at the front desk, the host asked him if he would care for rush service—even though Redd, Martin, and their small teams were the only ones in the entire hotel. Redd saw it as the host's effort to preserve a veneer of the mundane amid the chaos of an outbreak.

In the field, the CDC's role was to advise the District Health Management Teams, made up of Sierra Leoneans overseen by the Ministry of Health. Martin and Redd were clear that they were not in charge, but they were there to help.

In Tonkolili, Martin found the barest beginnings of an outbreak response; they did not even have a computerized list of where cases had been popping up. So Martin and the district team leader hunched over a map, marking villages where Ebola was present with a felt pen. The patterns that emerged informed the district team, which would be dispatched to identify cases and quarantine homes. Sometimes in the face of local reluctance, the district teams acted as detectives: freshly dug graves, an abandoned house, nervous villagers—anything that could be a sign of an Ebola case would raise suspicions and warrant further investigation.

Martin spent most of his days riding along with the district health team, sometimes two or three hours at a stretch to reach far-off villages. One day, they traveled to Masokori, a village north and east of Tonkolili's capital, Magburaka, to investigate reports of a suspected case. When they arrived, Martin watched an ambulance pull up—not to pick up the ill, but to return five survivors who had weathered Ebola's horrible storm at a treatment center in Kailahun. The survivors, all women, were met by joyful villagers who escorted them into town. Four returned, beaming, to their homes. But as if he needed a reminder of the terrible toll he was witnessing, Martin watched the fifth woman collapse, sobbing, on her doorstep. A member of the district health team told Martin that the woman had gone to the treatment center in Kailahun with her daughter. The mother returned. The daughter had not.

In Bombali, Redd spent most days hurtling between one crisis and the next. On October 21, his morning was spent at the local hospital in Makeni, where an eighteen-month-old boy had exposed most of the nurses to Ebola. Redd scrambled to find new nurses as the others quarantined themselves—nurses to take care of the nurses. Redd realized they might have to close the pediatric ward, another blow to Sierra Leone's already-weakened public health system.

When he returned to his headquarters, Redd called Jonathan Towner, a CDC lab technician based in Bo. Every day, blood samples would be ferried from Makeni to Bo, where Towner's lab would look for the telltale signs of Ebola's presence. Every day, Towner and Redd spoke by phone, ticking off the list of people who needed to be transported to a treatment unit, or quarantined at home.

On this day, however, something was odd: one of the tests had come back inconclusive. One of the indicators of the virus's presence had been triggered, but the other had not. That meant they had to test the patient again. Redd asked who the sample belonged to. When Towner read the man's name, Redd felt his stomach drop—the sample had come from a member of the district health team.

Redd found the team outside, gathered around their colleague who might have just received a death sentence. He had to get to the holding center at Makeni's hospital, where he could be quarantined while his blood was tested again. When they finally found an ambulance to take him, the rest of the team felt a sense of complete deflation. Many wept openly.

But slowly, another, more frightening realization set in: The man was their colleague. They had worked together, in close proximity, for days. If he had Ebola, the district health team, the CDC team, and the WHO officials in Makeni had all been exposed. Redd returned to the Wusum, his head spinning, worried about the effects of a close call on the district team—or even worse, an exposure.

That night, meeting with his fellow virus hunters at the hotel, Redd explained what had happened, from a safe physical remove. The night was sticky with tropical heat; the air conditioner had picked that day to shut down, and the atmosphere in the upstairs lounge where they gathered felt repressive and confining. They had to get the young man's blood re-tested, and fast. But in a cruel twist of fate, the person who usually transported blood from Makeni to Bo had been in a car accident and was now confined at the local police station.

Martin volunteered to make the drive the next morning. Until then, Redd and Tiffany Walker, an epidemiological investigator who had also had contact with the young man, would quarantine themselves in their rooms to wait.

The next morning, Martin and Redd showed up at the holding center at Makeni's hospital, where the young man had sweated through a sleep-less night. The phlebotomist who was supposed to draw the man's blood was late, so late that Martin himself began preparing to insert the needle. Once the phlebotomist arrived, he followed the careful procedures for transporting potentially contaminated blood—the blood flowed into a glass tube, which was placed inside a screw-top specimen container. That container was in turn placed inside a plastic box, lined with double polyethyl-ene liners. The box went into another, larger box, to add yet another layer of protection. They checked and rechecked everything they had done—and they realized they had put the blood inside the wrong kind of glass tube. A test from that kind of tube, one with a yellow stopper instead of one with a purple stopper, indicating a different kind of chemical regimen, might be inconclusive yet again. They told the phlebotomist to draw blood yet again. The technician let his irritation show.

Once they knew they had gotten the process right, Martin jumped into a car for the four-hour trip to Bo. Floor it, he told the driver. They made it in three. When they arrived, Towner and one of his colleagues met them at the door to begin the testing process.

By the evening, Martin arrived back at the Wusum, spent and mentally exhausted from worry. He stopped by Redd's room, just in time for the phone to ring. It was Towner: The tests had come back negative, the young dis-trict health team worker did not have Ebola. Redd and Martin didn't even bother to try to suppress the relieved flood of tears. They raced to the hold-ing center to get the young man out.

"We were often short on good news in those days," Redd said later. It was a small victory, but one they cherished—not least because they were the ones involved. "You had to have faith that the interventions we were doing were going to work. Because it sure wasn't obvious right off the bat."

The village-by-village surveillance collected by teams in Foya and Bong and Bombali and Tonkolili yielded data that filtered up the chain, from regional capitals to Monrovia, Conakry, Freetown, Geneva, and Atlanta. The data illustrated where the virus was spreading and where it might spread next. That sort of meta data collection was relatively new to ministries of health in all three countries, though it was critical to stopping Ebola's spread. Without that data, contacts could melt away into the interior's dense jungle, lost until they started a new hot zone of their own.

Collecting and analyzing data became a critical tool in fighting the Ebola virus. Just as retail businesses, tech companies, and even political campaigns were coming to rely on Big Data to better understand their customers and constituents, so too were humanitarians starting to use data science to understand what was happening around them. But even by September and October, the man tasked with collecting these data—Luke Bawo, the Liberian Ministry of Health's head of Ebola surveillance—struggled through charts and sheets submitted from around the country, many of which were riddled with inconsistent and misleading information.

One day in October, a tall Swedish man walked into Bawo's office, in room 319 of the Ministry of Health's expansive building. Hans Rosling was something of a celebrity in the global health community, a no-nonsense believer in the power of numbers, built after decades of experience responding to some of the worst tragedies in Africa. Rosling, the former head of the Karolinska Institute in Stockholm, is mobbed by fans when he attends prestigious gatherings like the World Economic Forum in Davos, and his TED Talks sell out in an instant.

But Bawo did not know who Rosling was until the Swedish professor introduced himself. He had canceled his lectures and his classes, Rosling said, to volunteer. Within twenty minutes, Bawo had given Rosling a desk.

The data Rosling found were a mess. Parents might give conflicting information about their children's ages to contact tracers. Complicated Liberian names might be transposed, making it more difficult to trace those who were infected, or double-counting cases that actually existed. When investigators in rural northern counties didn't find an Ebola case in a given village, they would enter a "0" on their spreadsheet. That zero suggested there were no cases in that village. Rosling preferred to leave those spaces blank: It was more accurate to say investigators had not found an Ebola case, he said, than to say there were no cases to be found.

Rosling overhauled the Liberian database and asked Ministry of Health officials to scrub the lists they did have of duplicate names. That allowed precious resources to be conserved for actual cases, rather than forcing investigators to chase after cases that did not exist. The Ministry of Health began tracking multiple sets of numbers: the number of reported cases, to be certain, but also the number of funerals being held in rural counties, and the number of calls made to emergency medical lines.

He also used his celebrity to request a grant from a major Swedish foundation, established by a family that had made its money in part from mining the very West African countries that now suffered. Funding for the grant came through within forty-eight hours. He and Bawo became fast friends, keeping tabs on each other over the next several months. At meetings with international NGOs, the Swedish epidemiologist sat on the Liberian side of the table. Every other week, Bawo would take Rosling with him to report to President Sirleaf and her cabinet on the state of the outbreak. Bawo had to force Rosling to take Sundays off. Rosling, unwilling to leave his work even for the holidays, spent Christmas with Bawo's family.

Even with years of experience, the climate in Liberia was the scariest Rosling had ever encountered. Alone in his hotel room every night, he took to listening to the speeches of Winston Churchill for inspiration.

Rosling had his own moment of panic one night, when he came down with a case of diarrhea. He skipped dinner and took his temperature every two hours as he wondered whether he, too, had come down with the virus. Still, he finished a nightly report he was working on. When he woke up the next morning, he felt fine.[2]

In the meantime, they worked feverishly to compile the new data. Embedded with the Liberian government, Rosling became deeply cynical about the international response, which he found weak and enfeebled. He reserved his harshest criticism for the World Health Organization, which he came to view as worthless at best, actively unhelpful at worst. He favored two American Army lieutenants who had been sent to help crunch numbers in Microsoft Excel; the Americans, Rosling thought, were much more reliable than the WHO. Rosling was also resentful of international media reports that portrayed Westerners coming to the rescue of helpless Liberians; in Bawo and others, Rosling had found a set of deeply competent, deeply committed Liberians who were saving their own country.

The results of spreadsheets over which Bawo, Rosling, and their team labored were eye-opening. The number of Ebola cases in Liberia was not increasing as dramatically as CDC projections suggested they could have, but the situation was worse than the government itself portrayed. More important, the data showed them where to look for the next front in the war against Ebola.

But even with the CDC's increased efforts and Rosling's best data science, the case curve continued bending north. By the beginning of October, more than 7,150 West Africans were infected with Ebola, and more than half of those cases had occurred in Liberia. The dead already totaled 3,330 people. By the end of the month, more than 13,500 people would be infected, and 4,900 had died. The world needed a more robust response.

T W E L V E

Deployment

AFTER AN EYE-OPENING VISIT to Liberia, Jeremy Konyndyk and Tom Frieden took stock of what they had seen. The three West African countries were trying, and failing, to come to terms with a disease that had infiltrated both hard-to-reach rural areas and crowded slums in major cities. The health care systems in Liberia, Sierra Leone, and Guinea were so overwhelmed that other diseases were going untreated. Pillars of civil society in all three countries were breaking down; markets were shut, schools were closed. The World Health Organization (WHO) was plumbing new depths of ineptness on a near daily basis, while the vast majority of nongovernmental organizations (NGOs)—with the exceptions of Médecins Sans Frontières (MSF), Global Communities, and a few others—had pulled up stakes. On returning to Atlanta, Frieden had called President Obama to describe his experiences, and how the United States should respond. He was, by his own admission, worked up by what he had seen.

The Centers for Disease Control and Prevention (CDC) had asked for volunteers to deploy to West Africa, and those volunteers were being trained as fast as possible. But even the rapidly expanding American response was becoming overwhelmed. Members of the United States Agency for International Development Disaster Assistance Response Team (USAID DART), supplemented by doctors arriving on an almost daily basis, were no match for a disease that was infecting hundreds of new people every week.

Back in Washington, Konyndyk and Frieden shared the recognition that they needed more—more people, more resources, more expertise. Their agencies had never dealt with an emergency of this scope and complexity. In the following days, they briefed Anthony Fauci, of the National Institute for Allergy and Infectious Disease, who had heard similar reports from his own staff who had been to Africa. Together, they realized that the full force and weight of the entire American public health care system might not be enough to contain the outbreak.

Over the next two weeks, Konyndyk, Frieden, and Fauci dreamed up what they believed an effective response would look like. They needed thousands of responders to quickly—and safely—build the infrastructure necessary to care for so many more patients. They needed to project a sense of security, both for the West African people and for the foreign NGOs with the experience to fight an outbreak. They needed a regimented process to train the thousands of health-care workers who would be required to provide that medical response. They needed, in short, to create conditions on the ground that would be conducive to a long-term medical response.

There was only one organization in the world that had the capacity to deliver the manpower, the training process, and the security necessary to create those conditions: America needed to send in the U.S. Army, the single greatest logistical force the world had ever known.

"The decision to call in the military was a recognition that they can deliver speed and scale to a degree that no one else in the world can," Konyndyk recalled later. "It signaled to the world that this is a big deal, at a time when, frankly, very few others recognized that."

Konyndyk, Frieden, and Fauci first raised the prospect of sending in the military to other senior officials at the National Security Council (NSC), and with the Defense Department. Almost immediately, the NSC began gaming out the enormously complex questions a deployment to West Africa raised: How would they define the Army's mission? What, exactly, would they be doing? If one of the troops got sick, how would he or she be evacuated? How and where, in the case that an American soldier actually died of Ebola, would the Armed Forces medical examiner conduct an autopsy on the body?

The Defense Department and Army general Martin Dempsey, chairman of the Joint Chiefs of Staff, was largely cooperative, the NSC and public health officials recalled. But Dempsey insisted that soldiers would focus on a narrow mission, to build treatment facilities, not to treat patients. Health-care agencies, he made clear, had their mission; the military would have its own. There would be no crossover between the two. Some at the National Security Council found that position needlessly inflexible. Others understood exactly why Dempsey wanted to draw such a bright line.

"The military was there to support the humanitarian effort, and they were constantly of the mindset of, 'Who are we working with, and how do we build their capabilities so this is a short-term military engagement,'" Shah said. Amy Pope recalled Dempsey's clear guidelines: "Our role needs to be well-defined, and our role needs to come with clear objectives and timelines."

Frieden thought otherwise. He had been led to believe by Department of Defense officials that the Army would be able to set up and operate field hospitals within thirty days of deployment, and then staff those hospitals to serve patients. But Dempsey made clear to Frieden and others that the Army would not be staffing hospitals with sick patients.

To Dempsey, just a year away from retirement, the rules of engagement would dramatically reduce the risk any soldier faced. The military was already stretched thin after more than a decade at war in Iraq and Afghanistan, and Dempsey had neither the interest in nor the desire to get bogged down in another deployment with no clear exit strategy. Before a single Army soldier touched down in Liberia, Dempsey wanted to know who or what organization would be rotating in to replace them after their short deployment. Before the first tree was felled or the first cinderblock set, the Army had a plan to hand off each of the facilities it would build to a specific NGO.

The NSC worried, too, about the possibility that an American might get sick. The positive message such a show of force would convey, both to Liberians and to the world, could be completely undermined if the outbreak reached the Army. Even a single soldier falling ill would be a massive public relations disaster.

The prospect of a Western responder falling ill had already scared away many nongovernmental organizations. To prepare for the worst case scenario, and to alleviate fears that were keeping both the Army and foreign NGOs out of West Africa, the Pentagon decided to open a new Ebola treatment unit, one that would be reserved for Westerners alone, near the airport in Monrovia. It would be run by the U.S. government—more specifically, by the U.S. Public Health Service, a team of medical professionals more likely to be deployed to poor rural regions and Native American reservations with limited access to health care than to a hot zone like Liberia.

Rear Admiral Scott Giberson, who headed the Public Health Service, and Michael Schmoyer, who had coordinated the response to the Ebola crisis until members of DART deployed in August, traveled to West Africa to oversee construction of the facility, formally named the Monrovia Medical Unit. The bland and beige half-dome oval tent where patients were to be treated would be surrounded by supporting tents full of laboratory equipment and beds for the Public Health Service personnel.

On their way to Liberia, Giberson and Schmoyer missed their connection in Brussels. After three days cooling their heels in a hotel near the airport, they arrived in West Africa to find a metropolis on edge. Few cars were on the road, even in the middle of what should have been a busy workday. Even simple human courtesies went overlooked: when they came across a woman who had been hit by a car, screaming for help in the road, a group of Liberians would not come within ten feet of her, for fear she might be sick.

But the Monrovia Medical Unit itself was a wonder in the middle of a country in desperate need of help. By the time Rajiv Shah, Konyndyk's boss at USAID, toured the new unit, it was the most advanced medical facility in Africa, capable of delivering nearly the same level of care that an infected patient would have received at Emory or the U.S. Army Medical Research Institute for Infectious Diseases (USAMRIID).

At a meeting of NSC principals held Thursday, September 11, top officials agreed to formally ask the Pentagon for a plan. Department of Defense officials had been working on that plan for a few weeks; they delivered it to the NSC the following day, a Friday.

At the same time, the phone on Brian Gentile's desk rang. Gentile, a stoic-looking colonel, served as deputy commander of USAMRIID, the Army's medical research laboratory at Fort Detrick. He is steeped in Army culture, more comfortable reading through a PowerPoint presentation than speaking extemporaneously. Now, a top-ranking general needed quick action. He needed Gentile and his team to train the units that would deploy to Africa on the president's order. And that training had to happen fast.

Two days later, Gentile's first teams of trainers arrived at Fort Campbell, Kentucky, home of the famed 101st Airborne Division. They deployed another team to a military base in Germany, where troops were already preparing to deploy. Others went to Fort Bragg, in North Carolina, Fort Leavenworth, Kansas, and Fort Bliss, on the border between New Mexico and Texas. Within just a matter of weeks, USAMRIID deployed on 38 training missions, teaching more than 4,800 military and civilian personnel how to protect themselves from one of the most deadly viruses known to man. Some trainers returned home to Fort Detrick, in Maryland, only to be sent off to another base to train even more soldiers and civilians mere hours later.

Training is an important part of USAMRIID's mission. Initially created to explore possible biological warfare agents, the institute now considers itself the U.S. government's 911 emergency operator. They are the first call when another government agency—the military, humanitarian workers, or any other outfit—discovers a biological agent with which they are not familiar. A hotline, staffed twenty-four hours a day by medical experts, exists to help those other agencies identify what they are looking at in the field. USAMRIID even trained the Armed Forces medical examiner on how to conduct an autopsy of an Ebola victim, under biosecurity level-4 conditions—moon suits and all—in case Dempsey's worst fears of an infected service member came true. With a plan in place and training already begun, the NSC presented President Obama with Operation United Assistance, the mission that would ultimately deploy 2,692 U.S. troops to Liberia and Senegal,[1] where a few hundred support staff were based. The first commanding officer on the ground would be Major General Darryl Williams, the head of U.S. Army Africa Command, based in Vicenza, Italy. The Pentagon would then deploy thousands more troops from a division stationed back home.

The White House wanted to announce the mission as quickly as possible. The perfect opportunity was right around the corner, on Tuesday, September 16, when President Obama was scheduled to travel to CDC headquarters in Atlanta. That visit would provide a perfect backdrop to highlight the extent of the American response, to send a message to international partners and to an increasingly nervous American public that the situation would be brought under control.

But the timing was tenuous. When Obama landed at Atlanta's Hartsfield-Jackson International Airport that morning, Williams was in the air, headed to Liberia from his base in Italy. A line in Obama's speech declared that Williams was already on the ground. But speechwriters made clear to Gayle Smith, riding a few cars behind the president as the motorcade zipped toward the CDC base, that they would cut it if it was not accurate. As Obama's motorcade drew closer to Frieden's office, Smith pressed a cell phone to her ear, connected with a Department of Defense attaché at Monrovia's airport, monitoring Williams's plane. Just as Obama pulled onto the CDC campus, Williams landed. The line stayed in Obama's speech—Williams "just arrived today and is now on the ground in Liberia," he said.

"Our forces are going to bring their expertise in command and control, in logistics, in engineering," Obama announced after touring the CDC with Frieden. "And our Department of Defense is better at that, our Armed Services are better at that than any organization on earth."

The speed with which the deployment came to fruition stunned even those who were pushing to make it happen. It had taken just weeks for a major military deployment to go from concept to execution. It was a testament, in the minds of senior NSC officials, to just how seriously the administration was taking the outbreak. On the day Obama announced the new deployment, the cost of the United States response crossed the $100 million threshold.

"I don't know that I've ever seen a high-level policy decision-making process that's moved as quickly and decisively as that," Smith said a year later.

The military's arrival hailed a new moment in the fight against Ebola. At the darkest hour, when the situation felt so desperately out of hand, the most powerful force in the world was descending on Liberia to turn things around. Sending in the Army, American officials had hoped, would serve as a "hope multiplier." Deborah Malac, the U.S. ambassador to Liberia, later recalled Williams's arrival as a turning point. The next morning, she told Frieden, it felt as if hope was in the air once again.

Williams's first order of business was to open an "air bridge," an intermediate staging base that could accommodate the thousands of troops and the tons of construction and medical supplies bound for the area. The base needed to be close by, but not in-theater; Liberia's infrastructure could not handle so much American military traffic. They settled on building a temporary base in Senegal, about 1,000 miles away.

As the first hints that the Army would be involved, Major General Gary Volesky did some quick calculus and concluded that he and the men he commanded in the 101st Airborne Division were likely to get the call. Of the Army's ten active-duty divisions, several were deployed to Iraq and Afghanistan, several more had just rotated home, and some were training to return to combat zones. One more was on permanent guard on the Korean Peninsula. That meant, if the Army was looking for thousands of troops to send to West Africa, they would probably turn their attention to the 101st.

"When the Ebola outbreak occurred and the president made that announcement, there were really three courses of action, and we were number three," Volesky said later. "It became apparent that the other two courses of action were not going to work."

Volesky had taken command of the 101st just a few months earlier, after the division returned from Afghanistan. They were scheduled to deploy back to Afghanistan the following year, and rotating back into the field earlier than planned would present a logistical challenge—and a strain on the families who had just welcomed their soldiers home.

In New York, Samantha Power was running her own set of traps. Power, a former journalist and human rights expert who served as one of President Obama's earliest foreign policy advisers, had become the American ambassador to the United Nations a few months before the first Ebola cases began popping up in rural Guinea. She and other senior members of the Obama administration's foreign policy cohort, including Secretary of State John Kerry and National Security Advisor Susan Rice, had watched with growing alarm as the international public health community had fumbled the initial response. Now, as the case count skyrocketed, Power set to work convincing her fellow delegates to the United Nations to take the strongest stand they possibly could. The Americans hoped to send a message to the rest of the world that Ebola was serious, and that if they did not stop the disease in West Africa, they would be fighting it at home.

After the devastating civil wars of the past several decades, the United Nations already had a peacekeeping mission in Liberia, dubbed UNMIL (United Nations Mission in Liberia). A similar mission in Sierra Leone had wound down a few years earlier. Rededicating those troops deployed in Liberia to the other two countries, and redefining their mission in the process, was not feasible. Instead, Power and her fellow ambassadors crafted a new resolution to go before the UN Security Council, one that would establish the United Nations Mission for Ebola Emergency Response, or UNMEER. The resolution passed unanimously just before the UN's annual General Assembly, when dozens of world leaders descend on New York. The timing helped focus the attention of assembled heads of state on the crisis at hand.

The resolution represented the first time the United Nations had declared a public health emergency.

"The gravity and scale of the situation now requires a level of international action unprecedented for an emergency," UN Secretary General Ban Ki-moon told the Security Council. The UN's top Ebola response coordinator, David Nabarro, WHO director general Margaret Chan, and a health worker from Médicins Sans Frontières briefed the council by video conference from Monrovia.[2]

Some in the American delegation worried that the UN, a diplomatic body that works at a glacial pace, might be unprepared to mount a quick and aggressive response. In what may have been a telling omen, the resolution passed the Security Council unanimously—but only after all forty-five delegates spoke in its favor.

Even before Volesky heard from the Pentagon, he tasked his top civil affairs officer, Lieutenant Colonel Ross Lightsey, with learning all he could about Ebola, about the situation on the ground in West Africa, and about the mission they were likely to undertake. Lightsey came back from a quick trip to Washington a few days later, armed with organizational flow charts showing the key players, from the White House to the United Nations to the Liberian government itself. Their mission, as Obama had defined it in Atlanta, would be to build Ebola treatment units (ETUs) across Liberia, train workers who would operate those ETUs, to set up laboratories capable of testing blood samples, and to support USAID, CDC, and other agencies, which meant ferrying them around the country on helicopters.

Army culture is steeped in visual symbolism, and some officers taking in his presentation took exception to one of Lightsey's slides, which showed the 101st's logo behind and underneath USAID's. Lightsey explained his graphical design. This was not a situation like Iraq or Afghanistan, he said, where the military would be in charge of the vast majority of operations. Their mission was to support USAID, the lead American agency operating in Liberia, to work through the U.S. embassy, and to work alongside the Liberian Army, which had close ties to America's own.

"Liberia is the center of gravity here. The U.S. Army is not the center of gravity. We don't own Liberia, we don't own this mission," Lightsey told those present. "This is not combat, like Afghanistan or Iraq, where we own it. This is a sovereign country, with a legitimate president, with a fully functioning Army, and we're in a supporting role."

Volesky nodded in agreement.

Senior leaders at the 101st spent three straight days learning all they could about the Ebola virus, a reflection that this mission was unlike any other they had undertaken before. They had an enemy, to be sure. This enemy, this virus, wouldn't shoot back at them, but they also wouldn't be able to see it. Like other Americans unfamiliar with all but the basics of the Ebola virus, the soldiers of the 101st had some preconceived notions.

"We didn't know anything about Ebola," Volesky said. "It made people think that there was a guy with Ebola hanging out of a tree like a zombie." The briefings from academics, Volesky said, "took away all that mythology."

Back in Liberia, Williams designated the Special Purpose Marine Air-Ground Task Force–Crisis Response, a rapid response team based at Morón Air Base, south of Seville, Spain, as the unit that would evacuate any exposed or infected troops. On September 26, Defense Secretary Chuck Hagel called Volesky to formally assign the 101st Airborne Division to Operation United Assistance. Hagel made clear that Volesky could take any support units he wanted—engineers, air support, and others, especially from

Fort Campbell—so that the 101st would be working alongside fellow soldiers with whom they already had a relationship.

In a sign of how dangerous their mission might become, the storied division was told to prepare for 10,000 active Ebola cases, according to an internal military document prepared after they returned home.

In the coming months, the Army would ship in thousands of troops, 400,000 Ebola home health and treatment kits, and the construction supplies to build 17 treatment centers in Liberia alone, at a cost of more than $360 million.

Williams and his team took medical precautions to the extreme. On one day, Williams later recalled, his temperature was taken eight times.[3] Several times, troops reported symptoms that might be associated with Ebola, like fevers and headaches. Each time, it was a false alarm.

Much of the military mission was about psychology, as well as logistics. The new treatment facility near the airport, and public promises to evacuate anyone infected and the military's presence, American officials said later, were both meant to lure NGOs back into Liberia. Though the Army never made any promise to protect foreign NGOs or Western responders, the mere fact that there were thousands of Americans with guns around helped assuage security concerns.

The NGOs "couldn't get enough responders because they didn't know that either medical evacuation or world-class treatment existed should they get infected," Shah said later. "Once we put that in place, both the Medivac and the unit [to treat Westerners], it became clear we would be able to take care of the responders."

Days after Williams landed, Major Tony Costello's phone rang thousands of miles away at Fort Hood, Texas. Costello had been in Texas, assigned to the 36th Engineer Brigade, for only a few months, after being redeployed from an assignment in Italy. After graduating from West Point, his fifteen years in the Army had included several deployments to Iraq and Afghanistan. Now, he was told, he would be deploying one more time, to Liberia, where he and his team of engineers would oversee an ambitious plan to scale up the nation's Ebola treatment capacity.

As the disease struck more people, Liberia needed the beds in isolation units to treat them. The Army, Costello was told, would be building seventeen Ebola treatment units across Liberia. It was up to his team to develop plans for those new units, figure out how to get them built, even in remote corners of a remote country, and supervise the construction. And he had two weeks at Fort Hood to plan before he would be on a plane to West Africa.

It was fortuitous that Costello had only recently returned from Italy, for many of the first Americans who hit the ground in Liberia had served with Costello in Europe. He set up conference calls introducing his team in Texas to his former colleagues from Italy in the days before they deployed. Together, the two teams went over blueprints of previously constructed ETUs, sent over by engineers at MSF.

Two weeks after he was told he would deploy, an advance team made up of Costello and four of his fellow engineers were on a plane. Though Williams's team was working on opening an air corridor, it had not been established yet. So while Costello had deployed to Iraq and Afghanistan in the belly of mammoth U.S. Army transports, this time he found himself crammed into coach class of a commercial airliner bound for Washington's Dulles Airport, then to Brussels, then to Dakar, Senegal. The first sign that something out of the ordinary was taking place came in Dakar, when the cabin crew who had flown with them from Brussels stepped off the plane. They were replaced by a special cabin crew that operated the short leg between Dakar and Monrovia, in order to limit the number of Brussels Airlines employees who might be exposed to Ebola.

If Costello needed another reminder of the foreignness of his experience, it came when the plane touched down at Roberts International Airport in Monrovia. The field reminded him less of a bustling international hub than of a tiny regional airport in the Midwestern United States. He didn't even see distance markers on the runway, signs that let a pilot know how much runway is left—and, hence, how hard to slam on the brakes. (Costello's team would eventually be the ones to install those markers, a few months later.)

The small team pushed their way through the chaotic scene at the airport until they found their liaison from U.S. Army Africa Command. The liaison guided them to their first lodging, a spartan complex called the Phoenix Apartments that sat next to the old American embassy. The building's plumbing worked. The power worked, sometimes. The lack of furniture meant the team had to set up cots on which to sleep, though none minded the barren trappings. They had to hunt for a safe place to lock up their nine-millimeter sidearms. In Iraq and Afghanistan, military barracks had arms rooms where weapons were kept under lock and key; there were no such rooms in Monrovia.

The next morning, a Liberian driver in a rented van picked up Costello and his men for the short drive to the Palm Spring Resort, where U.S. Army Africa Command had set up their headquarters. The hotel was a strategic choice: It sat just a few hundred yards from the Ministry of Health and Social Welfare's main building. Headquarters turned out to be the hotel's main ballroom, though it was crowded with so many organizers, planners, and logisticians that Costello and his team found it easier to work down the hall, in the hotel's restaurant. At least the restaurant had Wi-Fi; if they needed to print anything, they would walk back to the ballroom.

As the 101st Airborne Division arrived, Volesky formally took charge from Williams on October 25. His troops had been building a tent city at the Barclay Training Center, a few blocks from the National Museum and the University of Liberia. After years in Afghanistan and Iraq, what the military calls "mature theaters," troops had been accustomed to at least some creature comforts, like real bunks. In Liberia, the accommodations were much more spartan. They spent four days setting up tents and arranging water, toilets, and fuel supplies. Even after the base was established, they had no hot water in which to bathe. Though they were not in a war zone, the Army maintained strict rules about which service members could leave base, and where they could go. They didn't want anyone snapping photos of themselves in a market where bats and monkeys were sold as food. It was a risk of exposure the Army just didn't want to take.

At the same time, massive C-17s loaded with helicopters from Fort Bliss were landing at Monrovia's airport, illustrating the benefits of sending in the U.S. Army. No other organization in the world could move so many people, and so much equipment, so quickly. Within days, a functioning Army unit could be established anywhere in the world; in October, that anywhere was the middle of Liberia.

Lightsey, who had returned to the United States from Afghanistan only a few months earlier, found himself shuttling between a series of meetings, coordinating the Army response with the myriad other agencies already on the ground. His day started with an 8:30 a.m. status meeting led by General Volesky. From there, he would sit in on the Incident Management System meeting headed by Tolbert Nyenswah, or check in with the new UNMEER teams and the UNMIL. His staff of forty or so in the civil affairs office were scattered around Libeira, coordinating directly with more local groups running the on-the-ground response. From their base at Barclay, Lightsey gave Volesky a daily overview of all that was happening in Liberia, from updates on the upcoming elections to the latest aid proposals by WHO in Geneva.

Volesky made a habit of showing himself in some of Liberia's most remote corners. He traveled by helicopter, frequently with Ambassador Deborah Malac and top Liberian military officials. Lightsey's staff made sure the logistics on the ground were taken care of. At times, though, Lighstey reflected on the strange arrangements: Where American soldiers were not present, Volesky's security was at times maintained by UNMIL—which had a sizable contingent of Chinese Army troops. The sight of an Army general being guarded by Chinese troops was disconcerting, though it underscored the humanitarian nature of their mission. "It was rather unique to have them participate in that," Lightsey said later.

A week after arriving, Costello's team got their first assignment. They would be building an Ebola treatment unit in Buchanan, the coastal capital of Grand Bassa County, population about 34,000 and three hours by car from Monrovia, where the outbreak had begun to spread. A British rubber company had donated land next to a river about ten minutes from downtown. Though it was so close to town, the site was a jungle; a local construction company was already at work removing trees and leveling the ground. Costello would be in charge of a team from the 902nd Engineer Company, who deployed from Germany.

Soon enough, Buchanan made the furnitureless accommodations in Monrovia look cosmopolitan. They spent the first week living on the second floor of a warehouse near the forested site—it was the only nearby space that was covered by a roof. The team did not even have tents: someone had forgotten to add them to the unit's packing list. By the second week, when carpenters had built floors and a tent roof on the new Ebola treatment unit, the team simply moved in. It saved plenty of time in the morning, as the platoon of about forty people just rolled out of their cots and started working. Costello kept in touch with his superiors back in Monrovia with a BlackBerry, the only device that seemed to work in Buchanan. If he needed more supplies—he recalled having to order a specific type of roofing nail— he would send a message up north. His superiors would send someone to a store that reminded Costello of a miniature Home Depot, to find the right equipment.

Once the Buchanan facility was on track, Costello and his team deployed to more remote sites. They visited Tappita, a tiny town in northern Nimba County; Barclayville, the capital of Grand Kru County in the far south-east; and Sinje, in Grand Cape Mount County west of Monrovia, to build new ETUs. In all three cases, he was struck by a remoteness that defied anything he had experienced before: Costello's team had to helicopter in to Sinje, hitching a ride with the 1st Armored Helicopter Brigade on one of the choppers that arrived in the belly of a C-17. At other sites, the lack of infrastructure sometimes meant that the only functioning bridge across a river consisted of a few felled trees. Costello found himself calculating how much weight those trees could hold, and whether dump trucks dispatched to haul gravel to the sites would make it across. In Barclayville, one overloaded dump truck snapped a bridge it was crossing; the driver scrambled out of the cab, but the truck languished for hours, dangling over the river. The gravel was crucial to the overall sanitation of an Ebola unit. It allowed safer drainage, an added layer of protection between the unit and the water table.

Other units fanned out to build Ebola treatment facilities in Voinjama, in Lofa County, the epicenter of the outbreak in Liberia; Zorzor and Ganta, along the border with Guinea; Gbediah, in River Cess County; Tubmanberg and Bopolu, outside of Monrovia. Constructing a facility took thirty days of hard labor, transforming a patch of forest into a miniature city. Engineers would fell trees and level a site, putting down gravel to ensure proper drainage. They would then build wooden floors and walkways, on which would sit tents housing everything from bathroom and shower facilities to the dangerous hot zones where patients were treated. The process was similar, though less arduous, for the six diagnostic laboratories that would test blood samples across the country, built by Army and Navy engineers, to go along with the USAMRIID lab run by Randy Schoepp in Monrovia.

Soon, the soldiers settled into something approaching a routine, one marked by early mornings, late nights, and predictable hurdles. Water became a serious challenge. Because ETUs require so much water, both for patient care and hygiene, Army builders needed to make sure that every unit they built had access to its own well or water source. They didn't want the units to be pulling water from local populations; many villages had enough trouble finding sustainable water sources on their own. And they did not want to have to truck in water, an expensive proposition that wouldn't survive after the deep-pocketed Pentagon pulled up stakes.

But Liberia is not blessed with a plethora of well-drillers. The few that Costello's team could track down were jury-rigged contraptions that looked liable to fall to pieces at any moment. One of the more reliable contractors would show up with his driller attached to the pickup bed of an ancient GMC Sierra. Even getting that guy to show up everywhere proved a challenge. At least two of the Army-built ETUs were delayed in opening over problems with water supplies.

Monrovia reminded Costello and his men of Kabul, a dusty town with garbage strewn in the gutters. After several deployments to a war zone, Costello was used to taking precautions, and to carrying his sidearm. But he soon felt something different in Liberia, something more welcoming.

When they deployed, Costello thought he was walking into familiar, dangerous territory. "We were thinking the Iraq, Afghanistan model. 'We've got to have weapons,'" Costello recalled thinking. "But we really didn't have to do that. We're not fighting these people."

Costello, who grew up in Atlanta, found the Southern Baptist and AME churches familiar. So too were the cars, many of which had clearly been shipped over from home. A self-described car fanatic, Costello saw cars with Liberian license plates screwed over plates from Minnesota and South Dakota. He kept half-expecting to see an old Mustang convertible, his dream car, flash down the street—until he actually saw one.

The Army took seriously the concerns that Dempsey, chairman of the Joint Chiefs of Staff, had laid out: Costello and his team were only there to build facilities, not to treat patients; Costello himself never saw anyone

infected with the disease they were fighting. While more than a few soldiers came down with minor ailments, from headaches to high fevers to
regular aches and pains, not a single American solider contracted the Ebola
virus.

Around them, it was a different story. By the time Costello landed in
Monrovia on October 16, 8,973 people had been infected across the three
West African nations, and 4,484 victims of the Ebola virus lay dead.

THIRTEEN

Dallas

FOR YEARS, THOMAS ERIC DUNCAN languished, alone, thousands of miles from his family, the woman he loved, and the son he hadn't seen grow up.

Duncan had been one of hundreds of thousands of civilians who fled Liberia's deadly civil war in the 1990s, forced out of his own home and into a squalid refugee camp across the border in Ivory Coast. He had tried to start over, living with his brother in a tent. The two young men befriended the woman who lived in the tent next door, Louise Troh; Duncan fell in love. Amid the poverty of years in the camp, Troh and Duncan had a son, Karsiah, in 1995.

Everyone in the camp longed for a visa to the United States, a veritable golden ticket that held the promise of a new life on American shores, far away from the violence and poverty of the home they no longer knew. Troh and Karsiah won the lottery in the late 1990s; Duncan, who had never married his partner, was left behind. He spent another decade and a half in the camp, where he learned French, Ivory Coast's official language.

Finally, in 2013, Duncan, still yearning for a ticket to America, felt it was safe enough to return home to Liberia. He moved into an apartment and got a job as a driver for a FedEx contractor. Louise had moved to the Dallas area, where Karsiah had grown up as a promising student, a high school quarterback who won admission to a college in San Antonio.

Then, Duncan's luck seemed to change. One day the phone rang at the home of Wilfred Smallwood, the brother who had shared Duncan's tent in the refugee camp and who now lived in Phoenix: "I got my visa! I got my visa!" Duncan shouted, ecstatic.[1] His life seemed to be moving again; he and Troh would be married when he arrived, his son thrilled with anticipation at the prospect of seeing his father once again. Troh helped him book his plane ticket, from Monrovia through Brussels, then to Washington and on to Dallas.

In the days before his plane left, a young woman named Marthalene Williams needed his help. Williams, the daughter of Duncan's landlord, was pregnant. She was also sick. Duncan, the landlord, and the landlord's son piled into a taxi with the young woman, bound for Monrovia's main hospital, and the nation's largest Ebola ward. Duncan later said he believed she was miscarrying; he didn't know she had the virus that was raging through his country.[2]

But the hospital had no room. Like so many others who were suffering, Williams was turned away. They got back into the taxi, and Duncan carried her into her own apartment. Williams, her brother, and her father would all be dead within a few days.

On September 19, Duncan arrived at Monrovia's airport. Asked whether he had been in contact with anyone who had Ebola, Duncan said no. Whether his omission of the young pregnant woman was a lie or whether he truly did not know she was sick remains unclear. Either way, Duncan showed no signs of any disease; he boarded the airplane. By the next day, after layovers in two of the world's busiest airports, he arrived in Dallas on United Airlines flight 822.[3]

Troh was ecstatic. She drove Duncan home to their apartment in Vickery Meadows, a melting pot of a neighborhood in Dallas, a magnet for new arrivals from South and Central America, from sub-Saharan Africa, a mini United Nations deep in the heart of Texas.

Five days after he arrived, Duncan began to feel aches in his joints and shooting pains in his abdomen. He developed a fever. That night, at 10:00 p.m., Duncan drove the few miles to Texas Health Presbyterian

Hospital. A nurse took his temperature—103 degrees, well above normal—and asked whether he had traveled recently.

Texas Presbyterian was one of the dozens of hospitals across the country that had made initial plans in the unlikely case an Ebola patient walked through its doors. Just a week before Duncan had arrived, the hospital had run drills to prepare for a patient who needed to be isolated.[4] The Centers for Disease Control and Prevention (CDC) had issued an advisory to American hospitals on August 1, urging those facilities to be alert for anyone complaining of fever, stomach pain, joint aches, vomiting, or diarrhea. The CDC issued a follow-up alert on September 4.

Duncan told the nurse he had just arrived from Africa, though he did not specify that he had been in West Africa. But the staff seemed to miss the message; a doctor prescribed Duncan antibiotics and sent him home to recover.

Over the next three days, Duncan's condition worsened. By September 28, he could no longer get out of bed, so weakened by the constant tremors and emissions that taxed his body. That day, he returned to the hospital's emergency room in an ambulance.

By now, the nurses suspected they might be dealing with something never before seen in an American hospital. Sidia Rose, the nurse who first interviewed Duncan in the emergency room, wearing some protective gear, asked her patient again about his time in Africa, and whether he had come into contact with anyone who might have been sick. Duncan once again said no. The doctors treating him huddled: Duncan might have malaria, they guessed, or gastroenteritis, or a particularly nasty flu. Or, one speculated, he might have Ebola. Duncan lay in the emergency room for at least three hours before his doctors put him in isolation.

At the home of Sonya Marie Hughes, one of Dallas County's nine epidemiologists, the phone rang. It was a special line, a twenty-four-hour emergency hotline that hospitals are supposed to call when they suspect an outbreak of some dangerous disease. Hughes called her boss, Wendy Chung. Chung, in turn, called the CDC in Atlanta: Ebola, she warned, might have arrived in America.[5]

When Chung arrived at the hospital, she was shaken by Duncan's blood work. The patient's platelets were low, something that might be caused by an infectious disease like Ebola. He was not throwing up yet, and there was no diarrhea. CDC operators in Atlanta weren't worried yet, because Duncan had not attended a funeral before leaving Liberia.

Still, Chung needed to test Duncan's blood for the presence of Ebola—and fast. Only one agency in the state, the Texas Department of Health in Austin, was capable of running a test for such a rare disease. But the department's experts in Austin were not even sure how they were supposed to transfer the samples from Dallas, about three hours north by car. Finally, after conferring with an increasingly nervous CDC, they agreed to have it couriered south for testing.

In the hours that followed, Duncan's condition deteriorated, and Chung's fears grew. Overnight, the patient began exhibiting more violent symptoms. Isolation, no matter how delayed, had been the right decision.

On Monday, September 29, the CDC announced that a patient in Dallas was being tested for the Ebola virus. Results were due the following afternoon.

Texas Presbyterian's staff was quickly overwhelmed with the incredible amount of work it took to care for just one patient in isolation. Among the nurses asked to aid Duncan, fear was becoming palpable. But they knew their calling, and they stuck to their work. All were given the opportunity to decline to treat Duncan. None shied away. The precautions they took got progressively more restrictive: first, nurses wore only masks, then face shields, positive-pressure respirators, another layer of gloves. The hospital had no full-body biohazard suits equipped with respirators.

On Tuesday, Duncan finally confided in one of the nurses treating him. He told her about Marthalene Williams, the young woman who had died after he helped her to and from the hospital in Monrovia. Chung blanched when the nurse relayed the story. At least seventy-six hospital workers had been exposed to Duncan while he showed symptoms of the disease—including Chung herself. How many dozens more, including the five school-age children who lived in Troh's apartment and the three-person EMT squad who had brought him to the hospital, had been exposed?

After calling the CDC, now convinced that Duncan had Ebola, Chung donned as much personal protective equipment as she could find and walked into the unit where Duncan lay. She began interviewing him herself: Where did you go? Whom did you speak with, touch, come into contact with? Dallas's top epidemiologist knew she was racing the clock to trace Duncan's contacts, to prevent an outbreak on American soil.

At the same time, she knew she would have to monitor herself for signs of the disease for the next three weeks.

Hours later, the blood work returned, and the CDC confirmed Chung's worst fears. The man in the isolation ward had Ebola. A rapid response team, headed by the legendary epidemiologist Pierre Rollin, dispatched immediately from Atlanta. That night, an increasingly anxious state saw its governor, Rick Perry, holding a press conference at the hospital, trying to reassure his constituents that every possible precaution was being taken.

On Wednesday morning, Gary Weinstein, the doctor in charge of Duncan's care in the hospital's Medical Intensive Care Unit, reviewed his treatment options, slim though they were. A blood transfusion using blood from someone who had recovered and built up antibodies was not among those options. Neither Kent Brantly nor Nancy Writebol, the only two Americans with antibodies, matched Duncan's blood type. ZMapp, the drug that may have saved both of them, was not a choice either because the supply of the hard-to-create drug had run out. The CDC recommended against another drug, TKM-Ebola, which would probably have made Duncan even worse.

The only option, he concluded, was brincidofovir, an experimental drug that had never been tested in humans.[6] Manufactured by Chimerix, a North Carolina–based firm, the drug would stop the virus from replicating—if it worked at all. Even before they gave the drug to Duncan, hospital administrators would have to jump through a series of hoops, filing reams of paper required to grant what is called an Emergency Investigational New Drug Application with the Food and Drug Administration. (When news of the possible intervention leaked, Chimerix's stock rose sharply.)

Outside the hospital, in Vickery Meadows and around the neighborhood, Chung's team and experts from the CDC began tracking down everyone who might have had contact with Duncan. Initially, they believed that number might be small, no more than two dozen people. Eventually, they found more than one hundred people Duncan had been around—all of whom would need to be monitored for the next three weeks.

Though the CDC was in town, it quickly became apparent to local officials that the agency was not about to take over the entire response. Even if the CDC was equipped to take on such a mammoth task, they lacked the authority to do so. That hit home during a conference call, when Texas health commissioner David Lakey suggested establishing an incident command structure that would put one person in charge. Clay Jenkins, the Dallas County judge—the chief executive of local government—loved the sound of that idea.

"Well, who's going to be in charge?" Jenkins asked on the call.

Tom Frieden, the CDC's director, spoke softly: "You would be in charge," he told Jenkins.[7]

"Everyone thinks the CDC comes and takes charge," Lauren Trimble, Jenkins's top aide, later told a journalist. "That was our assumption. Well, they don't. They'll help, sure. But we still have to do it."[8]

Once the enormity of his task had set in, Jenkins began re-creating a response the county had executed a few years earlier, when a flu sickened hundreds around Dallas. The county set up an emergency operations center on the third floor of their building downtown. Their first job would be to take care of Troh's apartment.

The apartment itself posed the greatest immediate threat of spreading the disease. It was where Duncan had spent days sweating, possibly bleeding, possibly excreting other bodily fluids. They would need to sanitize the entire space, though those who had shared it with Duncan while he became more and more contagious would have to be quarantined. Troh's family, unable to leave the house, had to rely on donations from a local food bank.

Health officials dropped off fliers to residents at the Ivy Apartments warning about the dangers of Ebola and offering pointers on how to protect themselves. Many of the residents, though, did not speak English as a primary language, making it difficult to comprehend the fliers they had been given.

The county also needed to tamp down a growing sense of panic that was clearly infecting their populace. One of the young boys in the household had gone to school at Tasby Middle School on Wednesday; school officials had to send him home. The children in Troh's apartment attended four different schools; attendance at those schools plummeted from a daily average of 96 percent to 86 percent as nervous parents kept their children at home. Students told reporters waiting outside those schools that other children, the children of African immigrants, were being bullied.[9]

The panic was spreading, too, to other parts of the country—and with a month to go before American voters cast ballots in midterm elections, the public's reasonable fears were being inflamed for partisan gain. Perry established a state task force to combat infectious diseases and called on the Obama administration to create enhanced screening facilities for travelers coming back from West Africa, accompanied by fully staffed quarantine stations. Senator Jerry Moran of Kansas, who headed the Republican Party's Senate campaign arm, and Representative Frank Wolf of Virginia demanded that the White House appoint a single adviser in charge of the response to the outbreak. (They suggested three senior statesmen, Mike Leavitt, Robert Gates, and Colin Powell—all Republicans.) Senator Ted Cruz, the ambitious young Texas Republican, asked the Federal Aviation Administration what steps could be taken to prevent passengers potentially infected with the virus from coming to the United States.

Republican candidates running for Senate seats in North Carolina and Michigan began calling for a ban on travel between the United States and West Africa. Influential members of Congress in charge of committees that oversee commercial aviation agreed: "We believe a temporary travel ban for such individuals who live in or have traveled from certain West African countries is reasonable and timely," Pennsylvania Republican Representative Bill Shuster and South Dakota Republican Senator John Thune said in a letter to the administration. Representative Dennis Ross, a Florida Republican, introduced legislation to restrict commercial flights and travel visas for anyone from Liberia, Guinea, and Sierra Leone. House Speaker John Boehner said banning flights sounded like a good idea. (It did not seem to matter to any of those leaders that there were no direct flights from Monrovia or Conakry or Freetown to the United States; all passengers would have to connect through Lagos, or Brussels, or Paris, or London, and none of those countries had implemented travel bans.)

To humanitarian officials in charge of the response such as Anthony Fauci and Rajiv Shah, travel bans were exactly the opposite of what needed to happen. The flights were a lifeline, one that funneled medical responders into the places they were most desperately needed. Banning flights out of West Africa effectively meant banning doctors and nurses from flying into West Africa. They told President Obama that banning flights outright was a policy prescription that yielded no real results. During his first term, Obama had lifted a twenty-two-year-old ban on travel to the United States by those infected with HIV. At the time, he said, the policy was "rooted in fear rather than fact."

But to political strategists, a call to ban flights played precisely to the fears most American voters harbored. Soon Republicans calling for a ban were joined by some Democrats—including Senator Kay Hagan, locked in a tight race for reelection in North Carolina (one she would ultimately lose). Polls showed 41 percent of Americans had "not much" or no confidence in their federal government's ability to respond to the outbreak, including a majority of Republicans.

Only one Democrat, Arkansas Senator Mark Pryor, attacked Ebola from the other direction. He accused his opponent, Republican Tom Cotton, of voting to take funding away from disease fighters at the CDC. In November, Pryor lost by seventeen points.

Outside the political realm, others began acting more irrationally. Navarro College, a small two-year community school sixty miles outside of Dallas, sent a letter to several applicants from Nigeria on October 2, informing them that their acceptances had been rescinded because they lived in a country with confirmed Ebola cases. A teacher at a Catholic school in Louisville, Kentucky, quit her job rather than take a twenty-one-day paid leave after returning from a medical mission in Africa. Geographic logic had no place at Saint Margaret Mary Catholic School. The teacher, Susan Sherman, had served her mission in Kenya, on the other side of the continent from the infected countries.

Dallas County officials had contributed to the chaos, too: CNN had aired an interview with Louise Troh, in the days after Duncan was admitted to the hospital, in which she claimed that her family was being quarantined inside an apartment still crawling with Ebola-laden bodily fluids. Health officials realized they had not even figured out what kinds of permits they would need to transport debris from the apartment to an incinerator. Troh's family waited for days before health officials finally took away the sheets and towels on which Duncan had slept.[10] By Friday, Hazmat crews cleared out the apartment, stuffing everything but the walls into protective bags, and then into barrels. They had to chainsaw through the television and the PlayStation as Troh's family stood nearby, still in the clothes they had put on that morning.

Hours later, Jenkins had found a home for the family, thanks to Dallas mayor Mike Rawlings. Rawlings's son had vacated a house he was renovating a few miles away; to transport the family safely, and without scrutiny from the news media flying helicopters overhead, Jenkins made a call to the White House. Soon, those helicopters got an order to vacate the area; a dignitary, they were told, might be flying into nearby Love Field, so they needed to clear the airspace.[11]

The family spirited down a back stairwell, escorted by Jenkins into an idling SUV. It drove them the half hour to the new house, a small four-bedroom affair where the family could complete its quarantine out of sight of the media—and, importantly, in a safe, clean environment.[12]

In the hospital, Duncan continued to fight, and he tried to stay upbeat, though his body was failing him. On Tuesday, he asked doctors to play an action movie. On Wednesday, he told his nurses he was hungry—a positive sign that he might be staging a comeback. They fed him a packet of saltines and a can of Sprite, though he managed to take just a few sips.

The outward signs betrayed the extent of the damage the virus was causing. There was blood in Duncan's urine, and doctors began to grow worried about his lung function. By October 4, his condition was downgraded from serious to critical. His organs began failing, just as the supply of the experimental drug, brincidofovir, arrived.[13]

Two days later, on Monday, October 6, Duncan's mother, sister, and nephew arrived at the hospital, after driving all night from North Carolina. Doctors only allowed them to see the rapidly deteriorating Duncan through a closed-circuit television monitor. Finding her son glassy-eyed and virtually comatose, his mother Nowai Korkoyah dissolved into inconsolable sobs: "My son is dead!" she wailed.[14]

Nurses cared for Duncan around the clock. He was heavily sedated, tears running down his face. By Wednesday morning, his pulse had dropped to the mid-forties. The brincidofovir kept dripping through his intravenous, but doctors realized that their last hopes were diminishing rapidly. Duncan's blood pressure suddenly dropped, a terrible indication of what was to come. One of the nurses, John Mulligan, wiped the tears away from Duncan's eyes. It would all be okay, Mulligan told Duncan.

Fifteen minutes later, at 7:51 a.m. on October 8, 2014, Thomas Eric Duncan's heart stopped.

Jenkins and Troh's pastor made their way to the home across town a few hours later. They sat away from Troh, to avoid becoming exposed themselves, and told her the man she loved was gone. Troh lost it. Her son, Karsiah, had not been able to see his father before he died. The closest he came was signing papers allowing Texas Presbyterian to cremate the body.

Dallas County officials were not yet out of the woods. Still within the incubation period were 177 people who had come into contact with Duncan—friends, neighbors, children, and medical personnel. They checked their temperatures religiously, monitored by everyone from the county health department to the CDC in Atlanta. Every cough, every ache that would otherwise pass unnoticed became cause for concern.

It was a young nurse, one of those who had treated Duncan, who began to feel unwell first.

Nina Pham had a reputation for getting things right, for double- and triple-checking patient charts to avoid mistakes. The twenty-six-year-old daughter of Vietnamese refugees had earned her degree in nursing from Texas Christian University; friends there credited her with inspiring them, and even teaching them, to be better nurses. Just two months before Duncan had arrived, she had received her certificate in critical care nursing.

But on October 10, Pham developed a low-grade fever. She called one of Dallas County's epidemiologists to warn her; when Pham's temperature hit 100.5, she drove herself to her own hospital, where she was put in isolation just ninety minutes later. Jenkins and the epidemiologists were stunned at the news: Pham had not been on the list of those who might have been exposed.[15]

Doctors raced to treat her aggressively, assuming the worst. Three days later, the day after the CDC confirmed that Pham had become the first person to contract Ebola inside the United States, she received a blood transfusion from Kent Brantly; unlike Duncan, Pham's blood type matched Brantly's, and within hours Ebola-fighting antibodies were coursing through her veins.

On the same day, one of Pham's colleagues, Amber Joy Vinson, boarded a Frontier Airlines flight from Cleveland to Dallas. A Kent State graduate from the small town of Tallmadge, Ohio, Vinson, age twenty-nine, had returned to her childhood home to plan her wedding; she visited a bridal store to try on dresses while she was there.

During her time at home, Vinson had begun feeling unwell. Her temperature also began rising, to 99.5 degrees. The day after she arrived home, Vinson's fever went up again; it took about twenty-four hours for blood tests to reveal that she, too, had Ebola.

The fact that Vinson had traveled twice, from Dallas to Cleveland and back, alarmed CDC doctors, and spooked the media. Federal authorities raced to track down about 150 people with whom Vinson had come into contact in Ohio, including 87 people on the two Frontier airplanes she flew. (The airline took one plane out of service and replaced seat covers and carpet near where Vinson had sat.) A Transportation Security Administration agent in Cleveland, who had patted Vinson down on her return trip, was placed on a three-week paid leave. So were the six members of the Frontier flight crew, four flight attendants and two pilots, who flew from Cleveland to Dallas.

At the same time, another lab worker who handled the Liberian man's blood had departed on a cruise a few days before; when she started feeling unwell, the lab worker quarantined herself in her cabin until the cruise ship neared Galveston, Texas. Federal officials had already asked the governments of Belize and Mexico to allow the lab worker to disembark; both countries said no. Governor Rick Perry refused to allow the ship to dock with a potentially Ebola-infected person aboard, so the Coast Guard dispatched a helicopter to pick her up. She never developed symptoms.

There is an old and cynical saying in the news media: If it bleeds, it leads. Vinson and Pham quickly proved that blood need not be spilled to provoke a frenzy, much of it centered on rumors that proved inaccurate. Reports that Vinson had traveled against doctors' orders turned out to be false; she had been given approval to fly home by a CDC physician.

Still, the media publicly fretted about the prospect of so many who had come into contact with Duncan traveling freely across the country. Both Ohio and Texas implemented new rules restricting travel for anyone who might have been exposed.

In truth, the physical characteristics of Ebola make it susceptible to oxygen, making transmission unlikely, though not impossible. But calm and rational analysis of medical facts are tough to fit into a breaking news headline on television.

A debate was brewing, both on public airwaves and on the conference calls between senior medical officials, over how Pham and Vinson had been infected. No one knew for sure; neither nurse could remember coming into direct contact with Duncan's bodily fluids. The CDC's Frieden had seemed to suggest, the day after Pham fell ill, that the nurses had not properly protected themselves. He apologized a day later for seeming to blame the nurses for getting sick, though Frieden and Anthony Fauci continued to believe they had not followed protocols.

Duncan's infection, and the subsequent infections of Vinson and Pham, deeply shook the White House and those who believed that the U.S. hospital system was better prepared to catch any potential Ebola cases. "We all had the impression that any hospital would not only be able to recognize that somebody was infected with Ebola, but take appropriate precautions," said Amy Pope, the president's deputy homeland security adviser. "We had gone into it with the assumption that U.S. providers would be able to recognize the signs of Ebola."

Texas Presbyterian had missed those signs.

"Basically, the facts showed we were wrong on two counts: One, the hospital did not do the travel history [on Duncan], so they basically missed it the first time he was at the hospital. So they didn't recognize from the outset, so that made clear to us that we needed to put some other triggers in place," Pope said. "The second piece was, what kind of infection control did they exercise?"

The patients, Pham and Vinson, were lucky that their symptoms were caught early. Duncan had been sent home to fight the virus alone for three days. Now, hypersensitive to the possibility of Ebola's spread, doctors intervened the moment both women showed any signs of infection. And where the CDC had been caught off guard by Duncan, they were more ready to treat new patients—just not at Texas Presbyterian.

Only a handful of facilities around the nation are capable of treating a patient under biosecurity level-4 conditions: the Nebraska Medical Center,

Emory University in Atlanta, the National Institutes of Health (NIH) in Bethesda, Maryland, just outside of Washington, and the U.S. Army Medical Research Institute for Infectious Diseases (USAMRIID) at Fort Detrick. The Nebraska facility was already treating one patient, Ashoka Mukpo, a freelance cameraman who had contracted Ebola while on assignment in Liberia. The NIH offered to take Pham; she arrived in the Special Clinical Studies Unit, on NIH's Washington-area campus, on October 17, about a week after her first symptoms. Vinson would be sent to Emory, where she arrived on October 15, just a day after being diagnosed.

Instead of simply isolating patients, all four hospitals were practicing what they called "supportive care," an intensive treatment regimen aimed at keeping the body strong enough, long enough, to develop its own antibodies. Doctors worked hard to maintain vital signs like breathing and blood pressure, to ward off the hemorrhaging and organ shutdown that progressed during advanced stages of infection. Treating a patient with so much attention required an around-the-clock staff effort; in Bethesda, about twenty-seven people per week treated Pham.[16] In Atlanta, Vinson too received blood transfusions from both Brantly and Writebol.

Pham was most worried about her dog, a Cavalier King Charles spaniel named Bentley. A week earlier, a dog belonging to a Spanish missionary who was fighting for his life after returning from West Africa had been euthanized; health officials there were worried that the Ebola virus might lurk in the dog's blood and infect someone new. Pham did not want her dog to suffer the same fate. Jenkins, the Dallas County judge, was also determined to save the dog, for public relations purposes if nothing else.

Fortunately for Bentley, the U.S. Army Medical Research Institute for Infectious Diseases had an answer. The diagnostic tests that the Army scientists had prepared before American troops were deployed to Liberia would also indicate the presence of Ebola in dog blood. USAMRIID had run those tests in case the 101st Airborne had taken Army working dogs with them on deployment. (Ultimately, the military decided against taking their dogs.) Army doctors and veterinarians kept Bentley in quarantine for three weeks, testing his blood from time to time to see if he had picked up Ebola. The virus never showed itself in the dog.

Both Pham and Vinson, overseen by teams of dedicated doctors, recovered remarkably quickly. In just a week after arriving in Bethesda, five straight blood tests showed the Ebola virus had left Pham's bloodstream. Nine days after she arrived at Emory, Vinson, too, was declared virus-free.

Pham walked out of the NIH facility under her own power on October 24, two weeks after first falling ill. At a press conference surrounded by the doctors who treated her, Pham—showing no outward signs of the aftereffects of the virus—read a brief statement. Fauci, among those who had treated her, made a point to put his arm around her, to demonstrate there was no risk in touching a survivor. "She has no virus in her," Fauci said at the press conference. She was reunited with Bentley when she returned home to Dallas.

Four days later, Vinson, too, walked out of Emory looking healthy, if shaken. She wiped away tears as she thanked God, her family, and the medical team that nursed her back to health.

In Washington, with an election around the corner, Republicans began ratcheting up pressure on the White House. Privately, even Democrats were worried that President Obama's response was missing the mark. What the White House sought to convey was a president executing a calm and steady response, driven by science and not irrational fear and panic. What the public saw, more often, was an aloof executive detached from the rising panic his constituents felt.

Obama tried to make clear that he took the threats seriously. The day Pham arrived in Bethesda, Obama canceled out-of-town fundraisers for Democratic candidates in Rhode Island and New York. He also signed an order that gave the Pentagon the authority to call up National Guard troops, if needed, to fight the outbreak.

Publicly, the White House still projected outward confidence. Most strikingly, Obama hosted Pham in the Oval Office. A woman who had been diagnosed with the most dangerous virus in the world just two weeks prior was photographed hugging the president of the United States of America. The photograph led all three nightly news broadcasts. He called Vinson, too, when she was released.

Back in Dallas, what could have turned into the first full-scale outbreak of the Ebola virus in American history, perhaps miraculously, did not. Days went by, with Jenkins, Rawlings, and their staffs on high alert. The first potential contacts, those who had been near Duncan as he deteriorated, began to emerge from quarantine with no symptoms. After three weeks, all 177 contacts were clear.[17]

But while scientists were beginning to understand the Ebola virus more intimately than ever, Pham and Vinson presented a new mystery: Was it the fast treatment they received that helped them recover so quickly? Was it the antibodies they received through blood transfusions from Brantly and Writebol? Was it the focus on keeping vital signs at healthy levels, to give their bodies the time to develop their own antibodies?

The experiences of Pham and Vinson, and of Brantly and Writebol before them, had taught scientists one valuable lesson: Providing support, no matter how ill a patient, was worth the effort.

"The general dogma in our industry in July was that if patients got so ill that they required dialysis or ventilator support, there was no purpose in doing those interventions because they would invariably die," Bruce Ribner, medical director of Emory University Hospital's Serious Communicable Diseases Unit, said at a press conference. "I think we have shown our colleagues in the U.S. and elsewhere that that is certainly not the case, and therefore, I think we have changed the algorithm for how aggressive we are going to be willing to be in caring for patients with Ebola virus disease."[18]

What Ribner meant was: If the worst happens, we know how to treat the Ebola virus. It was an important message for the world, both in the United States and for nongovernmental organizations still trying to decide how to be helpful in West Africa.

But at the same press conference, Ribner betrayed just how much the medical community had left to learn about the virus that had now breached American shores. Asked why Pham and Vinson had recovered so quickly, Ribner admitted: "The honest answer is that we're not exactly sure."

That uncertainty bedeviled the White House. The government's confidence in its ability to prevent an outbreak on American soil had been deeply shaken, and now they wondered whether the military—already setting up Ebola treatment centers at breakneck speed on the other side of the Atlantic—might have to build similar facilities back home.

"Because our confidence was so undermined by what happened in that Dallas hospital, the fact that two health care workers became infected in the hospital, created a situation of, we really don't have that much insight into the way our hospitals do business," Pope said. "There was a question of, could there be other Dallas cases?"

FOURTEEN

The Ebola Czar

INSIDE THE WHITE HOUSE, President Obama was not happy. By early October, a little more than six months after the World Health Organization (WHO) announced Ebola's presence in West Africa and about two months after the U.S. government ramped up its own efforts, political pressure was rising rapidly. In Liberia, the Ebola virus had shifted from northern Lofa County south into Bong County, while the number of cases in Monrovia spiked to more than 1,000. Back home, Obama's aides had worked hard to convey the impression of a federal government that had a handle on the crisis and could protect the American public from danger. But with an election just a month away, that impression was not sinking in.

Opposition Republicans seized on two concurrent crises—the Ebola outbreak and the rise of the radical Islamic State terrorist organization in Iraq and Syria—to sow unease among the American electorate. Public opinion polls showed that voters were pessimistic about the direction of the country to begin with, a trend borne of a deep economic recession from which America was only just beginning to recover. Throw in a killer virus and a pack of thugs rampaging through the Middle East with designs on harming Americans, and voter anxiety began reaching new heights. For an incumbent party, that anxiety can translate into a rout at the polls.

177

Democrats held a narrow majority in the United States Senate, and party strategists tasked with preserving that majority warned the White House that anything less than an all-hands-on-deck response would cost them seats.

Already, Republican candidates, beginning in Michigan and North Carolina, started using the outbreak in West Africa to attack their opponents. Amplifying that message, Republicans in Congress criticized the Obama administration for being slow to react, and for taking what they characterized as a disengaged approach to protecting American lives. Slowly at first, then more rapidly, Republicans started calling for a total ban on travel between the United States and West Africa. Some Democrats, sensing the political danger, joined the chorus. (Virtually every Democrat who called for a travel ban lost their election bids anyway.)

The American response to the Ebola outbreak, both in the United States and in Africa, was anything but hands-off. But the impression the White House sought to convey—cool, collected, no panic—sometimes felt more blasé than Obama and his aides intended. They meant to demonstrate to the public that everything was well in hand, that the president was not panicking. It was an attitude that extended from the president himself, a cerebral man who depended on rationality and science to guide decision making, both his own and that of the emergency responders at the Centers for Disease Control and Prevention (CDC), the United States Agency for International Development (USAID) and the Pentagon.

It was also an attitude that caused Obama significant political grief throughout his two terms in office, from the eruption of an oil well in the Gulf of Mexico in 2010 to the rise of the Islamic State and the administration's perceived lack of response; sometimes the public wants to see their president get angry and take action. George W. Bush grabbed a bullhorn on a pile of rubble in New York City in the wake of the September 11, 2001, terror attacks. That was not Barack Obama's style.

Washington power circles were replete with stories about No-Drama Obama, a president in an egocentric town who wanted his top aides to put ego aside. During the Ebola crisis, Obama told his advisers again and again to be guided by science; he would handle the politics. His attitude struck people like Anthony Fauci, of the U.S. Institute for Allergy and Infectious Disease, as a welcome breath of rationality into the frenzied and irrational political arena. It struck others—increasingly those Democrats who had to face voters just a few weeks away—as maddeningly naive and out of touch.

So by early October, Obama asked his team for a new solution. The political pressure from Senate Democrats was mounting. Thomas Eric Duncan was dead, and two nurses who had treated him were infected. Airport workers in New York had gone on strike, mostly to protest working conditions, though they also cited the threat of an infected passenger spreading Ebola as he or she walked through customs. The White House needed some new way to approach the evolving crisis, one that would give Americans the sense that their government was taking swift and decisive action.

Two Republicans in Congress had suggested just such an approach—name one person to oversee the whole-of-government response to the outbreak. In Washington parlance, name an Ebola czar.

The two Republicans, Senator Jerry Moran of Kansas and Representative Frank Wolf of Virginia, recommended three people for the job: former secretary of state Colin Powell, former secretary of defense Robert Gates, and former Health and Human Services secretary Mike Leavitt. Their motives may not have been altogether altruistic; Moran led the Republican effort to reclaim control of the Senate, and all three people he and Wolf had suggested were Republicans.

Two were nonstarters: Gates had penned a blistering book scorching the Obama administration after he left the Pentagon, and no one in the West Wing wanted him back under their roof. Leavitt had been a top adviser to Mitt Romney, Obama's opponent in 2012; he was in charge of building a Cabinet in the event Romney had beaten Obama. The third was Powell, Bush's first secretary of state, who had endorsed Obama back in 2008, but Powell had been retired for a decade and showed no interest in coming back to Washington.

Instead, on October 13, the phone rang in a penthouse-suite office about six blocks north of the White House. Denis McDonough, Obama's relatively new chief of staff, was on the line when Ron Klain picked it up. Ron, McDonough said, stay by your phone this afternoon. The president is going to call.

Klain did not have the profile of Powell or Gates or Leavitt, but he was well-known among Washington insiders. He served as chief of staff to both

Vice President Al Gore, during the Clinton administration, and Vice President Joe Biden, during the Obama administration. He is known in Democratic Party circles as the best debate coach around; he had coached everyone from Bill Clinton to John Kerry to Barack Obama on how to take a punch, and give one back, when they confronted Republicans on stage. Biden's masterful performance against former Alaska governor Sarah Palin during the 2008 vice presidential debate—that was all Klain's work.

Outside of Washington, Klain is best known as one of the lead characters in the 2008 movie *Recount*, which tells the story of the neck-and-neck 2000 election, ultimately decided by a handful of votes—and a Supreme Court decision—in Florida. Klain, one of Gore's lead lawyers after the election, was played by Kevin Spacey. (The physical resemblance isn't exactly spot-on: Klain is ebullient and excitable. He is a bit larger than Spacey, with a round face and flashing eyes, and he has quite a bit more hair than the actor does.)

Though Klain had not been a member of Obama's original circle of trust, a cabal notoriously difficult to break into given that the president trusted few beyond those who had served him for years, Klain had ingratiated himself. As Biden's chief of staff, he had spearheaded oversight of the mammoth $800 billion economic stimulus package, passed in 2009. Any government project spending that much money would be a natural target for waste, fraud, and abuse; Klain and Biden had worked hard to ensure there were no headline-grabbing stories about wasteful or fraudulent expenditures, an effort that largely—and improbably—worked. Klain had been present at another key moment in the Obama administration's brief history, helping to convince a Republican senator to switch parties in 2009, a defection that led directly to the passage of the Affordable Care Act, Obama's most significant domestic achievement. He had been asked to serve as Obama's chief of staff in 2013, though he turned it down (McDonough got the job).

Now, Susan Rice, Obama's national security adviser, called Klain to lay out what the White House wanted from him. A few hours later, Obama called, too.

The president told Klain he had confidence in the team at the White House at the moment, but that they were stretched too thin. Rice was overworked, juggling Russia's intervention in Ukraine, the rise of the Islamic

State in Iraq and Syria, and a hundred other crises that would have warranted front-page headlines but for everything else going on. Lisa Monaco, Obama's top homeland security and counterterrorism adviser, also had too much on her plate. As a consequence, decisions that needed to be made quickly were being put off. The outbreak, and its interconnected parts, was complicated enough that the White House needed one point person to oversee the entire response. For all his work in politics and public policy, Klain had built a reputation as a master problem solver, making him the right person for the job. He would report to Rice and Monaco, though he would regularly brief the president himself.

"There was an implicit recognition that there were a lot of hard policy choices to be made, and that the pace of that decision-making needed to speed up," Klain recalled later.

Klain called McDonough back the following day: He was in. On Friday, October 17, the White House announced that their former adviser would come back to take over the response.

He would start a few days later—even the Ebola czar needed to pass background checks and a drug test before reporting for duty. In those intervening days, he met with many of the younger staffers who would work for him, to familiarize himself with the scope of the challenge ahead and the faces of those who would help navigate them.

An expert at crafting the winning debate soundbite, Klain believed the key to tamping down the growing panic around the country was to communicate accurately, and honestly. They had to build public trust, and part of that trust was to convince Americans they were getting the unvarnished truth. Klain and Tom Frieden, head of the Centers for Disease Control and Prevention, agreed early on that the White House would neither review nor approve any science-based pronouncements that Frieden's agency wanted to make.

That also meant recalibrating the message coming from Obama himself. In the early days of the outbreak, Obama had promised that Ebola would never come to American shores. Then Thomas Eric Duncan had arrived, and gotten two more people sick. Obama, Klain said, needed to assure Americans not that Ebola would never show up in the United States, but that if it did, the government would quickly find those victims and isolate them, for the public good. Some inside the White House argued with Klain that a firmer promise would do more for public confidence; Klain countered that providing assurances that were both unrealistic and untrue undermined the White House's efforts. Obama sided with Klain.

Klain first arrived at his office in the Eisenhower Executive Office Building on October 22. His office, EEOB 300, was larger than most others in the building; it was on the same floor as the rest of the National Security Council (NSC), but in a prime location overlooking the West Wing. He attended McDonough's senior staff meeting that first day, in McDonough's large conference room next to the Oval Office. Then his new team met for the first time, about sixteen people in all, including two strategists from the legislative affairs office, a communications expert, and a handful of NSC staffers. For hours, they built a matrix of issues they had to work through, both at home and in Africa.

On the domestic front, two significant issues were the top priorities: first, how would they treat travelers returning from West Africa, those most likely to have been exposed to the disease? How would those travelers be screened at airports, and how would health officials monitor travelers during the twenty-one days of the virus's incubation period, when they might develop an infection? Second, what would happen if someone else got sick? Where would that person go, how would hospitals prepare for his or her arrival, how would the CDC respond, and how would top government officials be kept in the loop? Both questions required input and buy-in from a host of government entities, from the Department of Homeland Security, which oversaw agencies that controlled travel from foreign countries, to the CDC and the Department of Health and Human Services, which worked with hospitals.

Klain's team had a different set of concerns about the response overseas: How many beds should the U.S. government, through USAID and the Army, build in Liberia? How would they track the disease in Africa, given the notoriously inaccurate numbers being issued by WHO? What role should American-run hospitals play in the broader battle against Ebola in Liberia? How would they go about testing vaccines and other possible treatments, given the medical ethical concerns involved? And how should they coordinate between the three West African governments and nongovernmental organizations (NGOs), as well as the British and the French, who were leading international recovery efforts in Sierra Leone and Guinea?

On its face, the scope of the outbreak and the government response appeared unmanageably large. Officials at Homeland Security were overwhelmed by the prospect of keeping tabs on thousands of passengers coming from overseas. Health and Human Services could not fathom training the nation's hundreds of thousands of medical providers.

But to Klain, the crisis management expert, the perception was out of whack with the reality. And the reality was much more manageable. On any given day, only about 2,000 people who had been in Liberia, Guinea, or Sierra Leone over the previous three weeks were in the United States. Sometimes that number dropped as low as 1,400; during the holidays, it rose to about 2,300. So the question was not how they would track 300 million Americans, only how to keep an eye on 2,000 travelers.

Managing the passengers most likely to have come into contact with Ebola was a matter, Klain said, of "figuring out the right end of the telescope to look through."

"When I got there, the perspective was, 'We're a country of 300 million people, we have 5,000 hospitals, we have 500,000 medical providers. How can we possibly manage this disease in this vast [country]?' If I had any insight, it was, none of that matters. There's only 2,000 people we need to manage at any given time. We are just going to focus on managing those 2,000 people and making sure none of those 2,000 people have Ebola," Klain said later. "I think our team took a problem that had really taken the federal government, racking it with being overwhelmed, and helped reconceptualize it as a manageable problem. It's 2,000 people. It's manageable."

What made the problem even easier was that, of those 2,000 people, about 85 percent lived or stayed in a very small number of places: the Acela Corridor, between Washington and New York; Atlanta; Minneapolis; Chicago; Seattle; and Los Angeles. Health and Human Services (HHS) did not need to race to train every ambulance driver and dentist in Tulsa or Tallahassee; they only needed to focus on a small number of hospitals in areas where an Ebola patient was most likely to walk through the door. Any possible Ebola patient would be sent to one of those few hospitals, which would be ready to handle them. Klain's team, guiding efforts by HHS and the CDC, began to identify and prepare at least fifty hospitals across the country to handle a possible Ebola patient. Those facilities, which would be designated ETCs, or Ebola Treatment Centers, had to be within fifty miles of 90 percent of the population of travelers who returned from West Africa.

"We're not going to let [the next] Thomas Eric Duncan walk into some hospital in Dallas again that's not expecting him," Klain said. "We severely limited the number of facilities where someone was going to encounter the medical system. . . . Someone with Ebola is only going to have 50 touch points with the medical system, and we're going to get those 50 places ready."

Even the question of finding, screening, and monitoring passengers could be broken down into easy-to-manage constituent parts. Instead of potentially exposing thousands of customs officials at every major airport in the country, the Department of Homeland Security (DHS) officials worked with airlines to funnel passengers from West Africa through five airports—John F. Kennedy in New York, Newark Liberty International, Atlanta's Hartsfield-Jackson, Washington's Dulles International, and Chicago's O'Hare International. That allowed DHS to focus its training on Transportation Security Administration agents, and to build sophisticated screening facilities, at just five airports, rather than fifty.

National security agencies that had been beefed up in the years after the September 11, 2001, terrorist attacks helped too: "Customs and Border Protection are getting information about where someone has traveled and who they are, well before they actually get to the port of entry," said Amy Pope, the deputy security adviser. "We kind of used that same model here." American officials knew who was entering the country from West Africa, even if those travelers did not speak up themselves.

Despite calls from Republicans—and increasingly from nervous Democrats—to quarantine those returning from West Africa, scientists like Frieden and Fauci argued strenuously against locking people up. The science, they said, did not merit such an extreme reaction; in fact, requiring quarantine would have had a broadly negative influence on the fight against the outbreak at large. At a time when so many medical professionals were needed in West Africa, erecting barriers to them coming home would have a stifling effect. Even Kent Brantly, finally making his recovery, testified before a U.S. Senate committee against blocking passengers or creating quarantines.

"What the science says is that if you can really stay on top of the people that have been exposed to Ebola and get them just as they're starting to get a fever, the risk of infection to other people is very low. So science said there was really no reason to quarantine people if they were asymptomatic." Klain said. "Obviously, there was a lot of anxiety, and science couldn't say there was zero risk of transmission of the disease, but putting in place measures that weren't needed to address remote fears could really have slowed the overall response—which, ironically, would have made us less safe."

Klain's days started at 7:00 a.m., when he would arrive at the White House after driving through the slowly stirring streets of Washington. By then, two reports were on his desk—one, a domestic situation report, would detail the number of passengers who had arrived from West Africa the previous day, the total number of travelers who were within the twenty-one-day tracking cycle, and progress toward the goal of establishing the fifty Ebola treatment centers. The other, an international report, detailed the state of the outbreak in West Africa, updates on what the British and the French were doing in Sierra Leone and Guinea, updates on the Ebola Treatment Units (ETUs) that the American military was building in Liberia, and how many patients were in each ETU.

Klain would then walk across the small alley separating the Eisenhower Office Building from the White House itself, to attend McDonough's 7:45 a.m. meeting. An hour and fifteen minutes later, he met with his team. The rest of the morning and early afternoon, Klain sat in on a rotating series of meetings, either in person or by phone with top officials in London and Paris, the American ambassadors in Monrovia, Conakry, and Freetown and the NGOs working so diligently on the ground.

In the afternoon, Klain would meet separately with his domestic team and his international team. Any interagency problems, issues of jurisdiction or stepping on toes, would be worked out through phone calls between Klain and the various agency heads. Together, Klain, Health and Human Services Secretary Sylvia Matthews Burwell and Homeland Security Secretary Jeh Johnson worked hard to maintain good relations. (Klain's tenure overseeing stimulus spending made him the right man for a job heavy on greasing the wheels of interagency cooperation. At his going-away party several months later, the CDC's Frieden offered a toast: "Before Ron came, it was a long painful process to get documents clear that had to be cleared across the interagency [task force]. After he came, it was no longer long," Frieden joked.) After a wrap-up meeting at the end of the day, Klain would spend his evenings writing policy memos that would find their way to Rice, Monaco, McDonough, and President Obama.

As if the constant stress of rushing from one meeting to the next weren't enough, Klain had to keep tabs on any possible Ebola case that emerged inside the United States. And though the White House was working hard to tamp down paranoia, every day at least a few possible cases emerged. Every time public health officials discovered a possible case, an e-mail raced up the chain of command, eventually to a small handful of top officials—among them Klain, Burwell, the CDC's Tom Frieden, and National Institutes of Health's (NIH) Tony Fauci.

Even false alarms could be instructive; each one taught the feds ways to tighten up their screening processes.

One traveler arriving at New York's John F. Kennedy Airport, bound for Minneapolis, scared Klain's team when he disappeared for three days, only to surface back in New York with a fever. It turned out the man had missed his connection, then visited a dentist to deal with a toothache. The dentist had performed an invasive procedure; his patient did not have Ebola, he had an infection at the site of the dental work. Still, the close call convinced Homeland Security to proactively monitor arriving travelers, to make sure they got to their destination so as not to lose them in the bustle of a busy airport.

Days later, another man who had recently traveled from West Africa arrived at a hospital showing possible symptoms of Ebola. The hospital was one of those certified to handle an Ebola case, but it was the smallest, least experienced Ebola Treatment Center in the country. Rand Beers, a senior White House counterterrorism adviser who had served as acting secretary of Homeland Security, called Atlanta's Hartsfield-Jackson International Airport to stop a commercial plane at the gate so a team from the CDC could get on board and fly to the hospital.

But when they arrived, hospital administrators didn't let the team in. They did not want the federal government interfering in their hospital. We know what we're doing, the administrators said.

While the CDC team cooled their heels in the hospital parking lot, Klain called the governor. Look, Klain said, I don't have any authority to order you to allow the CDC team in. But if something bad happens and four CDC experts were waiting just outside the front doors, do you want to take that political heat? The team was quickly shown into the hospital, though they determined that the sick man was another false alarm.

On one cold January night, Klain got a call at midnight: a woman had shown up at a California hospital that wasn't among those trained to handle an Ebola outbreak. She had symptoms very like Ebola, including vomiting and a fever. She told doctors she had just returned from her honeymoon to Guinea. What scared Klain the most was that the woman was not in the government's database of returning travelers; where had she come from? How had she slipped through the surveillance efforts?

Klain spent a restless night trying to answer those questions in his own head. But another question nagged at him—who spends their honeymoon in Guinea, at the height of an Ebola outbreak?

The next morning, arriving bleary-eyed at the White House, Klain found that his suspicions were well-founded. The woman knew she had been in an African country that started with a G. But she got the actual country wrong; she had been in Ghana. And her symptoms were easily explained too: She was pregnant.

In all, during the 130 days Klain oversaw the American response, he got more than 300 warnings of possible Ebola cases. Every one turned out to be a false alarm.

By the time Klain arrived at the White House, the Obama administration had already spent more than $350 million—most of it through USAID—to fight the outbreak. The Pentagon planned to spend $1 billion more. The legislative specialists in Klain's office got to work on a new challenge: convincing Congress to appropriate billions more necessary to fight off the Ebola virus, both at home and abroad.

The White House announced its new request on Wednesday, November 5, the day after Democrats suffered the election losses they feared. In a letter to House Speaker John Boehner—one of those Republicans who had called for a travel ban—Obama asked for $6.18 billion in funding, most of it to USAID and the CDC, and about half of which would be spent in

Liberia, Guinea, and Sierra Leone. With spendthrift Republicans in charge of the House, and having just won back the Senate, such an amount could have set off serious objections on Capitol Hill.

But the White House targeted a few key members of Congress: Senator Lindsey Graham, a South Carolina Republican who had built a career as a foreign policy expert, and Representative Jack Kingston, a Georgia Republican who would retire from Congress just weeks later, became critical players. Both warned the White House they could have trouble selling a bill that would spend so much overseas.

Even in an era of hyperpartisanship, some of the old rules of politics still applied. The legislative experts at the White House made sure funding was included for every state to stock up on basic preparedness items, and for equipment for emergency medical services teams that might have to deal with an Ebola patient. Every member of Congress, in other words, could claim credit for helping his or her state prepare for a possible outbreak. On the contrary, if Congress voted down a measure to fight Ebola and an outbreak did occur, suddenly the onus would be on those members who voted no.

Still, Klain, cognizant of the battles he had fought over the economic stimulus package in which every member of Congress, even those who voted against it, wanted money for their states included, was leery of creating what is known in Washington political circles as a Christmas tree—a piece of must-pass legislation on which members of Congress hang their own pet projects. Klain pushed back against members who wanted special goodies added to the bill, yielding for just one: The final package contained money that would help foreign countries establish their own versions of the CDC, long a top priority for Senator Tom Harkin, an Iowa Democrat who would retire at the end of the current Congress.

The combination of carrot and stick—the ability to claim results for a member's home state, coupled with the risk of doing nothing and owning political responsibility for an outbreak—focused Congress's attention. And while the White House didn't get all it wanted, on December 16, as one of its final acts of the year, Congress passed a $5.4 billion funding measure.

The White House and Congress had sent two messages: first, the American public had evidence that their leaders were doing something to protect them from a deadly disease. Second, and perhaps more important, foreign governments once again got the message that the United States was leading the charge. Money invested by the United States yielded billions more in international commitments, both to the West African governments themselves and to the NGOs working on the ground.

"It was critical in the international dialogue about the response in West Africa because we were able to dog other donor nations and other NGOs [with] the fact that we were putting a lot of cash up to fund these things," Klain recalled a year later. "Our money yielded a lot of money from other countries."

Spurring action, both at home and abroad, remained an urgent priority. On October 22, the day Klain began his assignment in the White House, WHO reported 9,911 confirmed Ebola cases. By December 17, the day after Congress passed the funding bill, that number had almost doubled: 18,569 Guineans, Liberians, and Sierra Leoneans had been infected.

FIFTEEN

Panic and Quarantine

EVEN BEFORE RON KLAIN arrived at the White House, the spread of the
Ebola outbreak in the minds of the American people had made that fate-
ful jump, from a far-off foreign problem to a perceived threat at home. Few
concepts are scarier than the notion of a virus, something so small it is invisible except under an electron microscope, capable of killing in the most
gruesome of ways, especially if, as Michael Osterholm had written in the
New York Times in September, that virus goes airborne.[1]

The White House, led by the cerebral and logical president, insisted
on staying out of the way of the scientists who had both the knowledge and
capacity to be able to stop the virus. But while those scientists had the
expertise necessary to marshal the greatest Army against a pathogen in the
history of the world, they lacked the diplomatic touch, the art of spin necessary to communicate with an already frightened and nervous public.

On October 16, Tom Frieden of the Centers for Disease Control and
Prevention (CDC) arrived at the Capitol complex in Washington, to give
members of Congress an update on American efforts to fight Ebola. By then,
the CDC had 139 staffers on the ground in West Africa, and more than
1,000 agency staffers had provided logistics, communications and analyt-
ics support, both in Atlanta and overseas. Three thousand U.S. troops were

on their way to Liberia, and hundreds of doctors affiliated with global non-governmental organizations (NGOs) were pouring back in. Still, Frieden said, the outbreak represented "the biggest and most complex Ebola challenge the world has ever faced."

Looking over his lectern, Pennsylvania congressman Tim Murphy, a Ph.D. psychologist whose public health experience included appearing on a Pittsburgh television station to offer medical advice and who had called the hearing, delivered his own verdict: "The math," Murphy said, "still favors the virus."

Klain and others understood that they were battling public psychology, as well as a virus. Humans are conditioned, they knew, to fear the new threat much more than the old, more common threat, regardless of any logic. When we hear about a shark attack off the Florida coast, or a terrorist threat against a major landmark, we are much more likely to fear that new threat than we are to fear threats that, statistically speaking, are much more likely to kill us. Humans fear the shark bite and the terrorist's bomb more than they do being hit by a car, even though a car is thousands of times more likely to kill someone than a shark or a terrorist—or, for an American living across a vast ocean from the epicenter of an outbreak, than the Ebola virus.

It is another trick of evolution, a mechanism that allows our brain to keep on living despite the threat of being hit by a car—or, thousands of years ago, being eaten by a bear or a tiger as we slept in a cave—without being consumed by fear, while at the same time adapting to and factoring in new threats.

In his office on the grounds of the National Institutes of Health (NIH) just outside Washington's borders, Anthony Fauci, director of the National Institute of Allergy and Infectious Diseases, understood the sentiment. It was similar to one he had experienced with the rise of HIV and AIDS, a virus doctors struggled to understand and the public began to fear. Fauci, who has treated more AIDS patients than almost any other medical professional alive, remembered the panic of the 1980s, as the epidemic reached its peak, when people worried they might get AIDS from going out to a restaurant in Greenwich Village, where a gay waiter might be the server. Someone had asked Fauci: Can I get AIDS from eating spaghetti? Fauci had seen a similar panic after envelopes containing deadly anthrax were sent to some news outlets and members of Congress, just weeks after the September 11, 2001, terrorist attacks.

In the midst of the AIDS epidemic, after the anthrax attacks and now again during the Ebola outbreak, Fauci made the media rounds, trying to convey that the respective threats of contracting a deadly disease—from a gay waiter in a restaurant, from handling one's mail, or from a traveler returning from West Africa—were entirely out of touch with the actual risk. Once again, Fauci was called upon to appear on the Sunday morning news shows, on cable news, and on major radio programs, where he was asked about the threat of contracting Ebola. His strategy, honed over decades of dealing with a panicky public, was to repeat himself, again and again.

"You have to respect the fear of people," Fauci told an interviewer at the Washington Ideas Forum in October 2014, at the height of the U.S. panic. "You can't denigrate it and say, 'Why are you afraid?' You've got to explain to [the public], and you've got to do it over and over."

The fear of contracting Ebola was, Fauci and Klain knew, entirely illogical. But logic and rationality are among the first victims in a dangerous situation, and both men understood they would have to factor in the public terror as they crafted their own response. Irrational fear was not even confined to those who didn't do this sort of stuff for a living. USAID director Rajiv Shah recalled having returned from a trip to West Africa in mid-October, landing early in the morning and racing to his office to take a quick shower. Shah headed to the White House for a National Security Council meeting, to share what he had seen on the ground. When he told his fellow emergency responders—including some of the same medical experts who knew the real risks—that he had just returned from the epicenter of the outbreak, several of those at the table physically recoiled.

Shah, Fauci, and, when he came on board, Klain found themselves on the same side of the next significant policy fight the administration faced. After successfully fighting off proposals to ban flights between infected West African countries and the United States, they now faced calls to quarantine anyone who had traveled to Liberia, Guinea, or Sierra Leone.

To those at National Security Council meetings, quarantines were just travel bans by other means: quarantining travelers meant quarantining returning volunteers, the very doctors, nurses, logisticians, and Samaritans who were most needed to fight the disease. And that was before the 3,000

American troops would rotate home—how would the military quarantine so many of its own for three full weeks?

The debate had only just begun when one of those volunteers, a young doctor with an office at Columbia University in New York, woke up with a headache.

Senior government officials would later be struck by the image of Craig Spencer, a young hip emergency room physician who never lost his liberal idealism, sitting next to Kent Brantly, a deeply faithful man who worked for an organization run by the evangelist Franklin Graham, in the White House. The two men were from entirely different worlds, but both had traveled to West Africa to fight for some of the most impoverished people on the planet. More than a few in the Obama administration saw the common ground Spencer and Brantly found as refreshing evidence that, in a deeply polarized political environment, Americans on both sides of the ideological spectrum were good and selfless.

In the middle of October, Spencer, age thirty-three, had returned from a tour of duty volunteering for Médicens Sans Frontières (MSF) in Guinea. He was exactly the kind of volunteer MSF needed, having worked in some of the most battle-scarred regions of Africa, in Rwanda and Burundi. But the deployment to Guinea affected Spencer more than his previous stints overseas, he wrote later.

"The suffering I'd seen, combined with exhaustion, made me feel depressed for the first time in my life," he wrote in the *New England Journal of Medicine*.[2] He slept for hours on end and withdrew from his friends. Even back home, he felt the same angst about shaking hands or making physical contact that infused daily life in Guinea. He worried most about infecting his fiancée; the twice-a-day ritual of taking his own temperature caused minor panic attacks.

Ten days after he returned to the United States Spencer woke up with the certainty that something was wrong. Despite another night of deep sleep, Spencer felt exhausted, and he had a fever. His breathing was too rapid to be normal. The thermometer showed his temperature was creeping up. Spencer quickly called New York City's public health department to report himself. In a way, he felt relieved: "Although my worst fear had been realized, having the disease briefly seemed easier than constantly fearing it," he wrote. Within hours, Spencer was admitted to an isolation unit at New York's Bellevue Hospital, with a temperature of 100.3.

That afternoon, October 23, was Klain's second day on the job. He was sitting in the office of Sylvia Matthews Burwell, the secretary of Health and Human Services, when both of their phones vibrated. It was the CDC, activating a warning system established to alert top officials when someone showed up at a hospital to be tested for Ebola. Both Klain and Burwell scrolled through the CDC's alert, which included a fact profile of the patient: physician, recently returned from Guinea, and more specifically from an area in Guinea with a significant outbreak, showing symptoms twelve days after his last possible exposure to the virus. Check, check, check. And Spencer's temperature was rising every hour. Double check.

Klain raced out of Burwell's office, making his way back to the White House to mount his first response, little more than twenty-four hours after taking the job. Klain called New York governor Andrew Cuomo, and Tony Shorris, New York City's deputy mayor, to share what he knew and hear their plans. He and Shorris were having maybe their third conversation ever; they had been introduced a few days before, through a mutual friend. Now the two of them would have to come up with a plan to prevent Ebola from spreading through America's largest city.

Fortune once again smiled: If any agency in America knows what it takes to fight an outbreak, it is the New York City Department of Health, which has decades of experience tracing contacts and performing medical surveillance—though maybe not in something as deadly or as scary as Ebola. Over the years, the agency had battled everything from cholera to AIDS to the spread of bedbugs.[3] Contact tracing, the key first step to bring an outbreak under control, was old hat for New York's frontline medical workers.

Interviewers spoke with Spencer almost immediately to build a timeline of his activities after returning home, so they could identify and track anyone with whom he might have come into contact. Spencer detailed his calendar: he had ridden the subway, of course (he was, after all, a New Yorker). He had gone bowling, eaten a meatball sandwich, ridden in an Uber. He was worried beyond words about his fiancée.

Spencer represented a crucial test of the administration's efforts to maintain an impression of competence. On one hand, treating Spencer effectively and watching him recover could give the administration the feel-good story it needed to show that the federal government was capable of handling whatever might come its way. On the other hand, if anyone else got sick, the downside risks were tremendous. The stakes were so high it forced a sort of clarity in the moment.

"That was the beginning and the end of our communications strategy," Klain recalled later.

> As far as I was concerned, the only thing that mattered was that no one else in New York get Ebola. If we could show in those hard first ten days that Craig Spencer could leave the hospital healthy, and that no nurse, or no person who rode the subway, or no person who got in an Uber, or no person who bowled, or no person who ate a meatball sandwich, or no person who lived in an apartment building with a nurse or a doctor got Ebola, that was the only communications strategy that mattered. . . . The thing that was going to be most effective in allaying public fears was to be able to say to people: Well, look, you saw it with your own eyes. Nobody got sick.

The media was obsessively reporting the story, wondering aloud whether Ebola could be transmitted in the subway, in the meatball sandwich shop, in an Uber. Several outlets reported Spencer's condition just hours after he was admitted to the hospital, even identifying him by name. It galled Klain that Spencer hadn't even had the chance to call his own mother to tell her before news outlets reported his illness. It galled him more that outlets reported that Spencer had a temperature of 104.1 degrees—a dangerously high level that would seem to indicate he had been sick, and contagious, for days. Somewhere along the way, two digits had been transposed: Spencer's actual temperature by that afternoon had risen to 101.4, still high, but nowhere near as dangerous as early reports suggested.

After hanging up with Shorris, Klain met Obama, chief of staff Denis McDonough. and Lisa Monaco, Obama's chief homeland security adviser, in the White House's Diplomatic Room. Obama, conscious that a new case of Ebola, after the nurses in Dallas, would create new calls for quarantines and flight restrictions, cracked a wry joke: "Well," he said, "this isn't going to help."

The only way Klain knew the White House could assuage a nervous public would be to ensure that no one else got sick. There were not many appealing ways to satisfy media outlets intent on running ever more shock-inducing headlines on their front pages and in their broadcasts. But there was that third audience Klain needed to satisfy, an audience whose buy-in the government needed in order to create a truly national safety net to detect the first signs of any Ebola outbreak, and one that had its own financial future to consider. These were the hospital administrators, those professionals who ran the major public health institutions in big cities around the country.

The administrators had seen what happened to Texas Presbyterian Hospital in Dallas, when Duncan fell ill. Patients avoided that facility in droves, a situation that grew even worse when nurses Pham and Vinson contracted the disease. Revenue collapsed. Klain needed other hospitals to agree to serve as Ebola treatment centers in the United States, a process that would require them to spend lots of money to build isolation units, train staff, and ultimately gain certification, but one that could also cost them if patients started to wonder whether the virus lurked somewhere in their doctor's office. Just as Klain needed to prove to the public that no one else in New York would get sick, he needed to prove to other hospitals around the nation that they would be well taken care of if and when a patient with Ebola arrived on their doorstep. And that meant showing support for Bellevue now that Spencer was sick.

The difference between the American medical system and that of the other Western nation most likely to have to deal with Ebola cases, the United Kingdom, illustrated the difficulties the White House faced. In the United Kingdom, the centralized health system meant that the government could designate one hospital to treat any patients who came down with the disease. It was not the hospital's choice, it was the government's choice. In the United States, the federal government had no such authority, either over state hospitals or privately run hospitals. It was up to Klain and his team to convince hospitals that it was in their interest to accept any patients who might show up presenting scary symptoms.

If something went wrong at Bellevue, Klain knew that the task of convincing other hospitals to treat Ebola patients would be all the more difficult. On the other hand, if everything went smoothly, Klain thought he could portray the doctors and nurses at Bellevue as heroes, piquing the interest of other hospitals that might want their own doctors and nurses to be seen in a similar light.

Making sure everything went well meant working proactively as much as possible. As Duncan lay in intensive care in Dallas, his blood samples making their way to Austin for testing, the CDC had waited crucial hours before deploying a team to help Texas Presbyterian. The CDC would not make the same mistake again: even before Spencer's blood samples came back showing he was positive for the Ebola virus, CDC advisers walked through Bellevue's front door.

Those advisers set about creating a support network around the hospital, training nurses and doctors alike in donning and doffing personal protective equipment and other protective measures. The last thing anyone needed was another sick nurse. The CDC team began running down a checklist of questions they needed to answer quickly: Treating anyone with a contagious disease, especially one like Ebola, generates a lot of waste; where would that waste go? How would it be treated? How would the hospital deal with public anxieties about their nurses and doctors? Landlords who owned apartments where some nurses lived hinted that those nurses could be evicted because of the risk they posed. Every one of those questions had come up in Dallas; in New York, the CDC wanted answers before questions turned to problems.

At the same time, Klain, McDonough, Monaco, and their teams kept adjourning to separate meeting spaces across the White House's sprawling campus to hammer out the administration's policies on returning health-care workers. How would a returning volunteer like Spencer be monitored, quarantined if necessary? Hundreds of American doctors, nurses, technicians, and others who had volunteered in West Africa would be returning home in the coming months, and debates raged over how strictly those who came home would be monitored. They kept Obama apprised of the internal debate throughout the weekend.

If Spencer's proactive decision to call public health officials at the first sign of trouble demonstrated the best inclinations of a hyper-aware volunteer cognizant of the danger he or she might pose to others, the way another young returning volunteer was about to be treated demonstrated the worst instincts of politicians eager to show their own leadership, however misguided. And it would illustrate to the White House, once again, the urgency of creating a policy that struck the delicate balance between protecting Americans and protecting individuals, between preventing an outbreak at home and providing the resources necessary to fight the disease in West Africa.

Kaci Hickox had already had a long day, or days, when she arrived at Newark's Liberty International Airport on Friday, October 24, the day after Spencer checked himself into the hospital. The flight from Freetown required a stopover in Europe, and after a month in the hot zone, the stress of a long trip weighed on her. She had volunteered at an MSF clinic in Sierra Leone, a clinic where staff did not bother to count the number of victims who had died; it was easier to count the smaller number who survived. On Hickox's first day in the clinic, she had asked one of her patients whether any of her family members had gotten sick; the woman told her that seventeen family members had died within the past two months. On her last night, Hickox gently fed Tylenol and antiseizure medication to a ten-year-old girl whose body shook with violent tremors. Hours before she boarded a plane home, Hickox watched the girl die.[4]

So Hickox may have had other things on her mind when she told the immigration agent at the airport that she was returning from West Africa. The young man steered her toward a secondary screening room, a windowless facility in the bowels of Newark's airport. There, over the next four hours, she was questioned by a parade of officials. She got the sense that some were accusing her of an unspoken wrongdoing. Others exhibited at least a modicum of friendliness, introducing themselves and offering weak smiles. Someone brought Hickox a granola bar and a glass of water when she asked. The nurse noticed that one of her interrogators, a man from the CDC, was scribbling notes in the margins of the official-looking form he was filling out; the CDC's form did not include enough space for all the information the man had to collect.

After four hours, as she grew increasingly frustrated with her detention in the claustrophobic space, a U.S. Customs agent used a forehead scanner to take her temperature, then smirked when the readout showed Hickox had a 101 degree fever. Hickox knew a forehead scanner would be thrown off by her flushed cheeks. The agent seemed as if he didn't particularly care.

But she had little choice other than to follow the agent to an ambulance, which drove her to University Hospital in Newark. She thought the fuss the agents were making was beyond overkill. Eight police squad cars escorted Hickox the few miles between the airport and a tent, set up outside the hospital as a kind of makeshift isolation unit. The two senior doctors who attended to Hickox were confused—they were told their new patient had a fever. An oral thermometer, far more accurate than the forehead scanner, pegged Hickox's temperature at exactly 98.6 degrees.

"There's no way you have a fever," one of the doctors told her. "Your face is just flushed."

Hickox was the first person to be subject to new orders issued the day before by New York governor Andrew Cuomo, a Democrat, and New Jersey governor Chris Christie, a Republican. Under those orders, any travelers returning through John F. Kennedy Airport or Newark's Liberty from West Africa who had contact with an Ebola victim would have to be quarantined for the full twenty-one-day incubation period. If passengers lived in New York or New Jersey, they could be quarantined at home, subject to twice daily check-ins with state medical personnel.

For Hickox, who lived in Maine, that meant an extended time in the tent, which had only a portable toilet and no shower. When she asked to be allowed to take a shower, after two days traveling from the other side of the world and seven hours in an unpleasant airport quarantine room, hospital staff gave her a bucket and a sponge. Instead of a clean change of clothes, Hickox was given thin paper scrubs. Even her cell phone barely got reception. Her situation did not change when her blood work came back the next day: she had tested negative for Ebola.

Christie, a bombastic figure known more for yelling at anyone and everyone who opposes him than for any actual policy achievements during his two terms as governor, maintained that quarantine was the right approach, even as he repeated a number of incorrect statements. At a press conference on Saturday, Hickox's first full day of quarantine, while campaigning for the Republican governor of Florida, Christie said the nurse was "obviously ill." (Not known for backing down or admitting fault in the face of facts, Christie repeated his misinformation over the following years, including in a nationally televised debate just days before ending his quixotic presidential campaign in 2016.)

The next day, a second test of her blood came back, this one also negative.[5]

Hickox had the presence of mind to mount a public relations campaign, with help from a few well-placed friends. "I am scared about how health care workers will be treated at airports when they declare that they have been fighting Ebola in West Africa. I am scared that, like me, they will arrive and see a frenzy of disorganization, fear and, most frightening, quarantine," she wrote in an op-ed for the *Dallas Morning News*,[6] placed through a friend who worked at the paper.

On Sunday, Hickox's cell phone worked well enough to call in to CNN, where she castigated Christie's diagnosis from afar. "First of all, I don't think he's a doctor," Hickox said of the governor. "Secondly, he's never laid eyes on me. And thirdly, I've been asymptomatic since I've been here."[7]

After hanging up with CNN, Hickox told hospital staff she wanted to see her lawyer. She had not shown any symptoms since arriving back in the United States, though it still took hours of wrangling and negotiations before she was allowed to speak with an attorney. By Monday, eighty hours after arriving at Newark, she was freed, allowed to return home to Maine. Some of the hospital staff, who agreed with Hickox about the danger of blanket quarantine policies, made a show of shaking her hand without wearing protective gloves.

Still, Christie and Cuomo had put even more pressure on the White House. On Sunday, Obama met with his Ebola team and senior administration officials—twenty-six people in all, including Vice President Joe Biden, the secretaries of Health and Human Services, Defense, and Homeland Security, Attorney General Eric Holder, and others. They had to walk the thin line between acknowledging the obvious threat and allowing scientists to do the work that would actually stop the disease's spread.

"The President underscored that the steps we take must be guided by the best medical science, as informed by our most knowledgeable public health experts," the White House said in a statement that day.

He also emphasized that these measures must recognize that healthcare workers are an indispensable element of our effort to lead the international community to contain and ultimately end this outbreak at its source, and should be crafted so as not to unnecessarily discourage those workers from serving. He directed his team to formulate policies based on these principles in order to offer the highest level of protection to the American people.

In plainer English: the White House did not want to take the steps Cuomo and Christie wanted to pursue. They would have to find a way to convince Americans that returning health-care workers would not start their own Ebola outbreak once they got home—without locking them in a tent outside a hospital in Newark.

Christie's office tried to spin Hickox's departure as a political victory. She would return home by private transport, Christie's office said, not by train or plane. Another Republican governor facing a tough reelection fight in November, Maine's Paul LePage, said his state would work with Hickox to quarantine her at home; Hickox had no interest in such an arrangement. After just a few days, a state court refused to grant LePage an order forcing the nurse to stay home. She took pride in going for a bike ride with her partner the next day. She never came down with the Ebola virus.

Still, underscoring just how much the American public feared the Ebola virus, polling showed that a vast majority of voters sided with Christie over Hickox. Eighty percent of Americans told CBS News pollsters they wanted anyone returning from West Africa to be quarantined. In New Jersey, just 37 percent of voters said they believed the federal government was handling the outbreak well,[8] and two-thirds said they approved of Christie's decision to quarantine the young nurse.[9]

Just two days after Spencer was admitted to the hospital, Samantha Power and her team boarded an Air Force jet, a modified 737, at Andrews Air Force Base just outside the Capitol Beltway. Power hoped to raise global awareness by showing up in West Africa. And her presence would be notable: she would be the first member of President Obama's Cabinet to set foot in the hot zone. She brought along reporters from NBC News, the Reuters United Nations bureau chief, and Evan Osnos, a staff writer at the *New Yorker*, to shed some light on what she saw as an undercovered crisis.

"It was an opportunity to demystify Ebola," Max Gleischman, Power's spokesman, recalled in an interview later.

Still, Spencer's illness scared the team, and as Christie and Cuomo implemented new quarantine requirements in New Jersey and New York, the team members questioned whether they should go. They were supposed to return home to New York, where Power had to go to work at the United Nations. What would it look like if America's ambassador to Turtle Bay were stuck in a quarantine tent the way Kaci Hickox had been? Ultimately, Susan Rice, Power's predecessor and now the president's national security adviser, signed off on the trip.

Power stopped first in Conakry, Guinea, then in Monrovia, Liberia, and Freetown, Sierra Leone. As she whisked between government ministries and American embassies, Power and her team were subjected to the same rigorous cleaning processes as an everyday West African: bleach baths for their shoes, guards armed with forehead thermometers, constant handwashing. At one point, Gleischman asked Power to slow down, so the NBC cameras could capture her undergoing the screening process.

In Liberia, Power saw firsthand just how vast the scope of the outbreak had become. There were signs everywhere, advertising the emergency number residents should call if they found a dead body, or if they suspected a friend or family member was ill. Inside the giant emergency operations center in Monrovia, detailed maps of the city covered the walls. Blue pushpins represented the locations of those who might be infected. Red pushpins represented bodies that needed to be picked up. Gleischman was struck by the sea of blue and the islands of red, scenes of death and disease in a tightly crowded city of a million residents.

After a quick trip back to Monrovia's airport, then across the country in an Osprey, Power visited a mobile testing lab run by the U.S. Navy in rural Bong County, near the heart of the initial outbreak. They visited an Ebola treatment unit—though they stayed far away from any potentially infected patients, cognizant that Cuomo and Christie still had quarantine orders ready to be imposed.

A day later, in Freetown, the magnitude of the outbreak appeared most evident—the city was a ghost town. At a soccer stadium the British military had taken over to build their own operations center, Power watched new medical trainees, about to be deployed into the field, dress in full personal protective equipment and jog around a track under the tropical sun, preparing for the intensity of treating patients in a hot zone.

Power made a final stop in West Africa, in Ghana, where she met with Anthony Banbury, the American who had been placed in charge of the United Nations Mission for Ebola Emergency Response, or UNMEER, at the new group's makeshift headquarters in an industrial park near Accra's main airport.

Banbury had been in charge of field support for UN missions across the world before taking over as head of the Ebola response. And despite his thirty years' experience at the UN, he made clear to Power and her team that he was frustrated. Amid piles of gear stacked to the ceiling, like some kind of Costco for public health, Banbury told Power he had been frustrated by the logistical hurdles he faced, and the pace with which help was arriving.

"The U.N. just isn't equipped to do these things quickly," Gleischman said later, summing up the consensus view among the U.S. delegation. "It's just not fast, and this was a time where speed was literally a matter of life or death."

Frustration with UNMEER's slow start soon trickled down to American and other international responders on the ground. Within weeks, high staff turnover at the UN agency convinced many that the new mission was doomed to irrelevance.

Power's last stop came in Brussels, where her U.S. Air Force plane parked at the far end of the tarmac for half an hour while medical personnel were summoned to check the Americans for signs of infection. Once cleared, Power hosted about twenty European ambassadors at the American embassy to the European Union. She was there to shake the cup, to ask for international assistance, and to deliver a message. Get engaged in the fight in West Africa now, she told the assembled ambassadors, before you have to deal with Ebola in Europe.

Arriving back home at John F. Kennedy International Airport, the delegation went through the same security screening that every other traveler from West Africa endured. Their temperatures were taken, they told interviewers who they had met and where they had gone, and they wrote down their contact information and that of their personal doctors. Michelle Nichols, the Reuters bureau chief, snapped a photo of Ambassador Power having her temperature checked in the security line. For the next twenty-one days, Power—or, on occasion, her assistant—called the New York Public Health Department to report her temperature.

The fear spreading across the United States was born in part from a gross miscalculation of the actual threat that everyday Americans faced. But even those who were cognizant of the threat, the volunteers and scientists who lived day to day in the hot zone, felt the stress of the risk they were taking.

Their environment, where every surface could be crawling with the world's deadliest virus, where skin-to-skin contact was prohibited, infused every waking moment and made peaceful sleep difficult to come by. The more intimately familiar they were with the virus, the more it could embed itself deep in their imaginations. Some feared touching armrests on the airplanes that ferried them home; for others, it took weeks to be able to shake a friend's hand, or even to hug a loved one, without an instinctual fear. The virus's incubation period meant twice-daily appointments with a thermometer for three weeks after returning home, another reminder of the danger they faced, even an ocean away from the hot zone.

Joe Woodring, the CDC investigator who deployed to Liberia's northern Nimba County in October, hoped his mind wouldn't play tricks on him as he returned to his Washington-area home. He landed on a Monday, and while he appeared perfectly healthy, his young daughter did not—she had a head cold. Just minutes after he hugged his family, Woodring's daughter let out an explosive sneeze, all over her dad. Woodring's eyes went wide as he looked at his wife—this is not good timing, he thought.

Three days later, on his second day back at his office at the National Center for Health Statistics, Woodring felt the uncomfortable beginnings of a fever. He had been the first scientist from his office to travel to West Africa, which made him something of a guinea pig for colleagues who might follow in his footsteps. And he felt it: Though he wasn't showing any symptoms, and he had had no contact with anyone who might have been symptomatic in recent days, some of those colleagues, even those with medical degrees, were avoiding him. They made clear, subtly and overtly, that they were thrilled to welcome him back—after his three weeks of self-monitoring were over.

Now, Woodring started to worry. He was almost certain his temperature was rising thanks to whatever harmless bug his daughter had passed on. But now he felt a headache, too. It could be nothing, he thought. Or it could be the first sign of an infection. Woodring couldn't find his boss around the office, so he sent a quick e-mail detailing his symptoms. I think I should go home, Woodring wrote. Seconds later, a response from his boss: Please go.

On the way home, Woodring called his wife. In a tone as cool and measured as he could muster, and one that certainly didn't match the worst-case scenario playing out in his head, Woodring explained what was going on. It's nothing, he assured her. It's just that head cold. But just to be safe, they agreed his wife would take their children to her mother's house nearby, just for the night.

Woodring took his temperature once again that night. It had edged slightly higher, north of 99 degrees, but it hadn't spiked dramatically. He called the Maryland Department of Health's special line, set aside for those who had reason to worry; once again, he explained his situation, and his symptoms, and asked their advice—at what point should he start to assume the worst? After a few minutes of consultations, they agreed that if his temperature hit 101.5 degrees, and if he developed any other symptoms—another headache, severe joint pain, diarrhea—he would need to go to a treatment facility capable of handling an Ebola patient, in his case nearby Walter Reed Medical Center. As the late afternoon turned to evening, Woodring worried, less about himself and more about what his case could mean for others.

"Oh my god, this is going to look so bad on CDC," he said to himself.

But as the sun rose the next morning, Woodring's temperature had subsided, down to a normal 98 degrees. He had not taken any Tylenol, which can mask a fever; this gave him more confidence that the readings his thermometer displayed were real. He was in the clear; his relieved wife and daughters came home that night.

He had learned a valuable lesson. When he came back from his second deployment, a month later, Woodring warned his family beforehand. If anyone is sick, even with a tiny head cold, dad was going to stay somewhere else for a while.

SIXTEEN

The Obama Phones

KEEPING TRACK OF HEALTH-CARE workers returning from West Africa, and deciding how to deal with any who showed symptoms, continued to vex the Obama administration, and the local governments in states and cities where those health-care workers lived. But Ron Klain knew that the greater threat of a potential outbreak spreading from West Africa to the United States would come not from the few dozen health-care workers, but from the hundreds of ordinary Guineans, Sierra Leoneans, and Liberians who made their way to the United States on a daily and weekly basis.

The paranoia being spread by some politicians, leading to calls for an end to flights from West Africa to the United States, was overblown, intentionally in many cases. They fed an angry and anxious public, serving the political interests of candidates running in November's elections. But the crassness of the politics did not alter the fact that there were between 1,500 and 2,000 people from the three countries in the United States at any given time. That presented policymakers with a real dilemma—how does a government track so many needles in a massive, nationwide haystack?

Transportation Security Administration officials, those who would greet West Africans as they arrived at the five hub airports across the country, represented the front line. Reports that landed on Klain's desk and on

Centers for Disease Control and Prevention (CDC) director Tom Frieden's desk showed that customs officials were taking temperatures of about
75 percent of travelers from West Africa who arrived in the country.
That 75 percent would then be tracked over the twenty-one-day incubation period, to ensure that they did not develop symptoms later, once they
had arrived at their destinations.

From a statistical point of view, screening three-quarters of the most
at-risk population was enough to make the odds of an outbreak erupting
on American soil very small. From a public confidence perspective, however, it was not good enough. Klain lived in fear that one of the 25 percent
who went unscreened would show up at a hospital with Ebola, which
would reignite public angst and calls for restrictive policies like travel bans,
which would ultimately impede the response and cost lives. Statistical
anomalies, after all, are not easily explainable to the public in the age of
Twitter and cable news.

"I understood, and this is where I will not apologize for a certain amount
of politics coming into the process—politics not in terms of partisan politics, but politics in terms of understanding how public perception was going
to react to this—that having 25 percent of the people unfindable was unac-
ceptable," Klain later recalled. Better record-keeping raised the number of
those they could track to 80 or 85 percent, but still the margin for error
was too high. "We couldn't lose people," he said.

The increasing prevalence of cell phones and smartphones made the
administration's job marginally easier. Many travelers could simply give
their phone numbers to government officials, who would then call to
check in for the next three weeks. But a growing number of West Africans
were arriving with cell phones that did not have the right SIM cards,
which meant the phones would not work outside of their home countries.
Klain and others racked their brains, trying to figure out how to track those
without working phones.

Outside the White House, some businesses raced to fill the void. Mark
Penn, the longtime political strategist who had guided then-Senator
Hillary Clinton's presidential campaign against President Obama in 2008
and who had moved to Microsoft, called Klain one day to pitch his own
solution: the Fitness Tracker, a wearable device similar to a FitBit. Penn
said Microsoft would donate the Fitness Trackers, free of charge, to take

temperatures of those coming in from West Africa. The data would be relayed back to public health officials, who could use the information to spot a potential Ebola case early in the process.

Microsoft sent the devices to CDC headquarters for testing, but two problems nagged at Klain and Frieden: first, the device took temperatures well enough for general health assessments, but not precisely enough for medical purposes; that imprecision could lead to false positives—or, worse, false negatives.

Second, Klain was not thrilled with the idea of the U.S. government slapping a wristband on people who arrived from specific countries, especially at a moment when a growing number of fringe groups were warning about the federal government overstepping its bounds. "It felt a bit like, do we want the government putting bracelets on everybody?" he said. It wasn't even clear that wristband technology would be effective. Ultimately, the administration passed on Microsoft's offer to help.

At the beginning of November, Frieden had another idea, one that would toe the critical line between perceived government inaction and overreaction—why not give travelers entering the country from West Africa a temporary cell phone? That would allow health officials to keep track of travelers entering the country, while at the same time representing a relatively minor expense; there were only about seventy or so travelers from affected countries arriving in the United States every day, and cheap cell phones—burner phones, in popular parlance—would not cost that much.

More important, it worked: The CDC started a pilot project using the phones at one of the five airports just days later, demonstrating that handing out phones to West African travelers, recording the numbers, and then calling those travelers a few times a day could increase response and coverage rates to 98 or 99 percent. The phones virtually eliminated the margin for error that kept Klain worried.

But Klain had survived the first several years of the Obama administration, when conservative critics lobbed all kinds of loony theories at the White House to paint them as big-government socialists determined to redistribute wealth. One of those rumors early in the administration had centered on "Obama phones," a program that allegedly handed out free cell phones to low-income minorities and welfare recipients. Conservative websites like the Drudge Report highlighted those free phones as more evidence that the administration was favoring the poor, and predominantly minorities, over whites and those who paid their own way.

In truth, there was a new program that helped low-income Americans get cell phones, though the administration had little to do with it. A decades-old program known as SafeLink helped subsidize phone services for those with low incomes, in order to expand access to 911 emergency lines. The program is funded by telecom companies, rather than tax dollars; in 2008, during George W. Bush's presidency, those telecom companies expanded the program to cover cell phones and about an hour of airtime per month for Americans lowest on the economic spectrum.

But explaining decades of telecom history to conspiracy theorists—especially those who already believed Obama was born outside the United States, among other more far-flung tall tales—was futile. Klain could foresee the headlines that a new program to hand out phones to travelers would generate. "Great," he thought ruefully, "Obama's giving free phones to everyone from West Africa."

In the Oval Office, Klain and Frieden told Obama about the phones. They could drastically improve response rates, and quickly, but it would open them to a political attack. "Our opponents can say Obama's giving free phones to people from West Africa," Klain told the president. Obama laughed; he was not immune to the criticisms leveled by the conspiracy theorists. He promised to take the political heat if the phones became an issue, and told Klain and Frieden to get the phones to airports.

But even by November, nearly a year after the outbreak began in Meliandou and three months after the American government began to engage in a serious way, money was an issue. Obama had asked Congress to appropriate several billion dollars to the fight, money that would cover everything from the military's deployment to Liberia to provisions for hospitals back at home. Yet Congress had spent most of October campaigning ahead of the midterm elections. A formal proposal was slow to form; some Republicans did not want to spend more money without cutting other programs out of the budget. (The bill that eventually emerged was a bipartisan affair, albeit one that appropriated less than Obama wanted. Some Republicans, including South Carolina Senator Lindsey Graham and

Georgia Representative Jack Kingston, worked closely with the White House to pass a funding measure.)

The government procurement process added another layer of red tape. Contracts of any substantial size had to be opened to public bidding and internal review, a process that could take weeks or months. Frieden, especially, warned of the consequences of getting bogged down in layers of bureaucracy that came along with operating the largest government in the world. "Every day that we spend planning," Frieden told associates, "is a week we lose in the battle. There is no time to plan."

This was not a new problem for Frieden. Often, the CDC had faced tight timelines that were not conducive to the standard open procurement process. To get around those pesky rules, the CDC always turned to a long-trusted partner, the private CDC Foundation and its president, Charlie Stokes.

The CDC Foundation had been created by Congress specifically for the purpose of moving things along. Since its inception in 1995, the foundation had served as a repository for donors who wanted to assist the CDC itself, in support of the various crises around the world. Over the previous twenty years, the foundation had spent some $620 million backing up CDC operations in places like Haiti, devastated by an earthquake, and Indonesia, smashed by a massive tsunami. They even helped in New York City; the day after the September 11, 2001, terrorist attacks, CDC planes stocked with needed supplies purchased by the foundation were the only nonmilitary planes in the skies over the Northeastern United States. CDC rescuers working the Twin Towers told the foundation they needed computer batteries and satellite phones, so that's what the foundation bought.

Stokes, the only chief executive officer the foundation had ever had until his retirement in January 2016, had been in regular contact with Frieden. When the CDC director returned from West Africa in August 2014, Frieden had called to warn Stokes that the CDC would probably need the foundation's help again. The situation on the ground was bad, Frieden warned Stokes. "I think he had a sense early on that he would need the flexible funding," Stokes recalled of those early conversations.

Now, Frieden called Stokes again, with a specific request: We need you to buy thousands of disposable cell phones to keep track of the travelers coming back from West Africa. Stokes, on vacation in Missouri, stepped out into a driveway to take the call on his own cell phone. He apologized to his hosts, then spent the rest of the weekend researching where to buy so many phones. Stokes settled on Walmart. Within days, 4,654 phones were on their way to Africa, thousands more to the five U.S. airports where travelers from West Africa would arrive. The giant and oppressive rules governing procurement for federal agencies did not apply to Stokes's foundation; he just wrote the check.

Once the phones arrived at airports in New York, New Jersey, Chicago, Atlanta, and Washington, every traveler entering the country from West Africa went through the same process: CDC employees would take down a traveler's phone number and e-mail address; if they didn't have a phone that worked inside the United States, they would get one of Stokes's disposables. They also got a thermometer. Twice a day for the next three weeks, the travelers would call their local health departments to report their temperatures. Stokes, who traveled to all three countries a few months later himself, got a firsthand look at how the procedure worked as a backstop: When he came home, he forgot to check in for a few days. The CDC sent him an e-mail, reminding him to contact his local health department.

Stokes and Frieden had been thinking through ways to use the foundation's independence for months. While they could realistically rely on a handful of corporate partners to write big checks, Stokes knew from years of experience that most philanthropists like to hear how their money is spent, and that the bigger and sexier a project was, the more likely a donor was to give again—even if what a disaster relief effort really needed was some decidedly unsexy set of supplies, like body bags or paper towels. In Liberia, the Swedish data wizard Hans Rosling was experiencing the same thing. There were plenty of donors to go around, but those donors wanted to make sure their money was being spent prominently.

"All of the international organizations wanted their piece of the cake, and they wanted their piece of the cake to look beautiful," Rosling said. "Being on the Liberian side, this was our main headache. No one was bad, no one was evil, it was just that urge to show what my organization had done."

Stokes worried that the need for mundane equipment and supplies might scare away or bore some donors. But he began seeing signs that a new type of philanthropist was gaining prominence, a generation born of the tech industry, one that cared more about data and effectiveness than prominence and stature.

Frieden's first request of Stokes was to find donors to build new emergency operations centers in each of the three affected countries. The structures would represent a massive and lasting contribution: they would act as data centers, hubs for multidisciplinary teams that could direct resources on the ground to their most efficient targets while analyzing both local and national-level data. Nothing similar existed in Sierra Leone, Guinea, or Liberia; putting everyone under one roof, the thinking went, would dramatically improve the efficiency of operations.

But they were not cheap. Each center would cost an estimated $3 million, so Stokes needed to find $9 million. He spent an early fall weekend calling potential donors, coming up mostly empty—until he reached Paul Allen.

Allen, one of the original founders of Microsoft, has spent hundreds of millions of dollars over the years on philanthropic causes. He told Stokes he was interested in funding the emergency operations centers. Stokes initially misunderstood—he thought Allen wanted to fund one complete center. No, Allen told him, he would write a check to build all three. When costs spiraled, raising the total price by about $3.9 million, Stokes called back to apologize; would Allen like to cover the cost of just two of the emergency centers? Again, Allen told Stokes, he would write a check to cover the higher, total cost.

The finished products were massive, like huge gymnasiums, built by the same prefab contractor the foundation had used in Haiti. When Stokes visited the emergency operations center in Freetown, Sierra Leone, he found more than a hundred people hard at work, divided between critical teams. Some were British military, others CDC staffers or World Health Organization (WHO) officials. Ministry of Health staffers worked side by side with their international partners. British officers and members of Sierra Leone's army stood shoulder to shoulder in front of maps, flat-screen televisions, and tablet computers. Outside, backup generators hummed. In a nation where just 1 percent of the population has access to the Internet, the emergency operations center, built with a tech billionaire's money, buzzed with connectivity.

In one corner, a team of operators manned a series of phones. Surveillance teams, armed with some of the cell phones Stokes had purchased from Walmart, would call in to report suspected cases of Ebola or dead bodies that needed to be carefully contained. The operators tapped information into a specially created computer program that prompted all the right questions: Who was the victim? Where, exactly, was the body? Who lives nearby who we can call to learn about the family or the neighborhood? Once answered, the operators would call an ambulance or a hearse to pick up the victim.

Nearby, another team mapped the cases the operators charted. Walls covered in white boards and local maps showed the locations of any suspected or confirmed cases, an effort to plot the spread of the disease and, hopefully, get ahead of it. Every night at 9:00 p.m., the heads of each team met to report on their daily progress.

In Guinea, Stokes visited an emergency operations center in the basement of the only significant Western-style hotel in Conakry that offered reliable Internet access. It seemed like a nice facility. But the power cut out three times; at 11:00 p.m. on the night of his visit, Stokes found himself stuck in an elevator between the first floor and the basement. He was worried he would have to spend the night cooped up between floors.

It was clear that the officials Stokes was helping to pay for had spent many nights in the hotel basement. When he visited in January, a dismal Christmas tree sat neglected in a corner, weeks after the holiday had come and gone. Family photos adorned the walls.

In the field, the foundation funded smaller satellite centers. Stokes visited Bo, a regional capital about three and a half hours east of Freetown, where the CDC had built a lab center in a ramshackle government building. Even here, far from the country's largest city, the Internet worked, and backup generators thrummed as centrifuges spun. The once run-down building now hosted a high-containment laboratory, where blood samples were processed in metal shipping containers. Stokes was baking in the heat; he could not imagine what the lab technicians, decked in head-to-toe personal protective equipment, must be feeling.

Samples arrived seemingly all the time, flown in by United Nations helicopter and carted in on the backs of motorcycles. Once in the hands of lab technicians, the samples would be sprayed with chlorine, then opened. The paperwork associated with the blood samples would be laid out on the sidewalk, and sprayed with chlorine. Finally, the sample itself would be rushed into one of the containers for processing.

The connection between far-flung villages and the laboratory in Bo, and similar lab outposts across all three countries, largely relied on men on motorcycles. Ranging across three nations with dismally poor road systems, the motorcycles could reach even the most remote and isolated villages, dodging mud pits that would have consumed a car, zipping down forest tracks too narrow even for a small vehicle to navigate. If a sample that reached the lab tested positive—and by the fall of 2014, it seemed there were few samples that were not testing positive—the operations center could dispatch an ambulance to transport the patient, or the body, to an Ebola treatment unit or a morgue.

But Sierra Leone, Guinea, and Liberia are desperately poor countries, with desperately little infrastructure—and desperately few vehicles, motorcycles or not. Frieden told Stokes they needed to shorten the time between a blood sample being taken and a blood sample reaching the lab. That meant more motorcycles, and that meant reaching out to more donors.

Stokes found another set of donors who had made their money in the burgeoning technology industry, and who were now looking to give much of that money away. This time, it was Mark Zuckerberg and Priscilla Chan, the founder of Facebook and his physician wife. The couple wrote a $25 million check—one of the largest individual contributions the foundation had ever received—with shockingly few strings attached. Do what you want with the money, Zuckerberg and Chan told Stokes. Just tell us how you spent it afterward.

So Stokes dramatically increased the number of vehicles tooling around the rural communities of West Africa. The Facebook money bought 206 Toyota pickup trucks, so many that Toyota had to make a special shipment. Before the ship arrived, the foundation arranged to deliver many of the new pickups by airlift. The four-wheel-drive vehicles would allow ambulance teams to get in and out of remote villages, even during the rainy season, when torrential downpours could turn rural roads into frothing mud baths.

Stokes used more of the money to buy four hundred new motorcycles to spread between the affected counties in all three countries. Those motorcycles cut the time between when a patient showed symptoms and when his or her diagnosis came back from a few days to a few hours. "These guys were amazing how quickly they could cover these distances," Stokes said.

They saved lives, too. Early treatment dramatically improved the survival rate of Ebola patients and, just as important, isolating a patient before they spent several days showing symptoms could save their family members, too, and stop the spread of the disease.

Stokes also visited a small community centered around a palm oil farm, where a once-vibrant market now sat dormant. The CDC Foundation had supplied tents used to quarantine those with Ebola before they could be transported to a proper treatment unit. The market had once been the lifeblood of the community; now, food and water were being trucked in whenever the roads were passable. A CDC staffer manning the quarantine tents pointed to one of the motorcycle riders who helped bring samples in from far-out villages. The motorcyclist had not been paid in two months, the CDC staffer told Stokes; the CDC was giving him as much food as it could, so he could feed his own family.

Zuckerberg and Chan publicized their gift, and therefore the CDC Foundation itself, in a post on Facebook. Allen, the owner of the Seattle Seahawks, flashed advertisements to donate on the Jumbotron during home games. For a foundation used to handling a small number of seven-figure checks from corporate partners and major philanthropies, the huge number of small-dollar gifts that started to roll in almost overwhelmed their system. Ten dollars here, a hundred dollars there—they had never handled contributions on such a scale. Many of the most prominent charities in the country began sending larger contributions. The Robert Wood Johnson Foundation wrote the first million-dollar check of the campaign. The Bill and Melinda Gates Foundation contributed, then the Silicon Valley Community Foundation, an important gateway to big tech money.

Henry Schein, the company that makes personal protective equipment, donated money and gear; the hospital firm HCA wanted to donate beds, so Stokes directed them to the U.S. military. Johnson & Johnson wrote a seven-figure check, too.

Stokes thought that building the foundation's credibility was key to keeping the money spigot on. In normal circumstances, the CDC Foundation would take a percentage of each contribution to cover its own internal operations, like paying the rent on its Atlanta headquarters or paying the salaries of its employees. With the Ebola outbreak raging, Stokes suspended that overhead charge. Instead, he took $1 million out of the foundation's reserve fund to handle overhead.

In Africa, the speed with which the foundation could move impressed both government ministers and other nongovernmental organizations alike. The CDC's central emergency operations center in Atlanta could request money for some specific project. So could leading CDC officials in each of the three West African countries.

When a team of health ministry workers in Sierra Leone planned to mount a massive campaign to conduct door-to-door surveillance in a particularly hard-hit neighborhood, they asked the CDC Foundation for a grant of $160,000 to hire and train 400 staffers. The request hit the foundation's inbox on a Thursday; within two hours, the money was wired to the appropriate accounts. By Sunday, the 400 newly trained staffers were canvassing the neighborhood.

"A need could arise one day and be approved that day, and we would move funding that week, sometimes that day," Stokes said. During his January visit, a top CDC aide based in Sierra Leone stopped Stokes to tell him about the door-to-door canvassing effort, and the money that made it possible. "It literally blew our minds," the official told him.

As a side effect of the foundation's spending spree, the group was able to funnel some money to residents whose businesses had effectively been shut down by the spread of the disease. Accountants, lawyers, merchants, university instructors, and students, all of whom had seen their livelihoods vanish as society pulled inward on itself, were suddenly put to work driving vehicles or manning phone lines. To speed the purchasing process, the foundation partnered with eHealth Africa, a nongovernmental organization that had built an emergency center to track polio in Nigeria with

CDC Foundation money. On the ground, eHealth had the foundation's permission to buy what it needed to run the operations and lab centers, including everything from generators and fuel to water and toilet paper.

The flexibility in spending brought a measure of order to what had been a chaotic response. Officials with different organizations, whether the CDC or WHO or local health ministries, would wake up each day with a new idea about how and where to spend money. Priorities changed on a daily, sometimes hourly, basis. No government purchasing process would have been able to keep pace. But the foundation, not beholden to any particular set of rules, could dash off a check when a need arose, without marching through a procurement process.

"There are some emergencies for which even a nonprofit with flexibility like us still needs that extra step of unrestricted money. I don't think there will ever be a way for government to fill that gap," Stokes said later. "The typical grant-making process would not have worked here. There was no time for that."

In just a few months, as the U.S. Congress dithered over whether and how to fund the fight against the deadliest disease known to man, the CDC Foundation raised and spent $55 million—eleven times what they had raised to help Haiti recover from its earthquake.

Today, the emergency operations centers in Conakry, Freetown, and Monrovia are still in operation. The once-temporary facility in Freetown is now permanent, and bulked up with a new second story that houses permanent offices for CDC officials, who help train disease detectives to look out for other viruses that plague the populace.

But the emergency operations centers represented just one front in the war on Ebola. In the rural counties well inland from the crowded capitals, another front was opening up, one that would ultimately bend the deadly curve of an out-of-control virus down, for good.

SEVENTEEN

The Burial Teams

IN LIBERIA, GUINEA, AND SIERRA LEONE, the Centers for Disease Control and Prevention (CDC) Foundation had built groundbreaking new facilities to track the spread of Ebola. Médecins Sans Frontières (MSF), the World Health Organization (WHO), and a few other nongovernmental organizations (NGOs) were on the front lines in Ebola treatment units, battling to save the lives of those who dared to seek treatment. But health officials knew they were seeing only a fraction of the real picture. In three nations where Internet access was virtually nonexistent and major highways could be rendered impassable by a monsoon, they knew they were likely missing hundreds of cases, and hundreds of dead bodies that threatened to infect new victims. The CDC estimated that just 18 percent of Ebola patients in Liberia were being cared for in hospitals at the height of the outbreak.[1]

Those who did not find space in hospitals, or did not seek out treatment, were largely in rural counties far from Monrovia and Freetown and Conakry. They mostly constituted members of rural ethnic groups, still skeptical of central governments hundreds of miles away. They were those least likely to have access to modern hygiene, most likely to continue the traditional burial practices that put them in the closest contact with virus-laden corpses, and the least likely to voluntarily go to a medical facility run by their governments, or foreigners in space suits. Ebola's race through metropolitan West Africa represented the greatest threat of the virus spreading, but if health officials neglected the outbreak in regional capitals and even small villages, it would live to spread again, like a fire that has found new fuel.

The traditions of the tribes that dominated rural West Africa are replete with superstition and tales of magic. Secret societies carry out rituals deep in the jungles. Villagers believe they can curse a neighboring tribe, or, if some ill wind befalls them, that they have been cursed. It is vitally important that a dead relative be cared for, washed, and dressed for the afterlife once they have passed away.

That tradition in particular put villagers at special risk. Because an Ebola-infected body carries the largest viral load at the time of death, coming into contact with that body is a particularly dangerous endeavor. At the height of the outbreak, the World Health Organization estimated that 70 percent of new Ebola cases came when someone had contact with a dead body, and 20 percent of all deaths were caused by unsafe burial practices.[2]

Far away from Monrovia, three Liberian counties just south of the border with Guinea had been particularly hard-hit by the outbreak. Piet deVries, the senior country manager for Global Communities, had seen Bong, Nimba, and Lofa Counties up close, during his years in Liberia. They had suffered deeply during the civil war, and now they were suffering again, as equipment and badly needed medical gear piled up in the far-off capital.

After the civil war, Global Communities had been the first nongovernmental organization to venture back into Liberia. Since 2004, the group had been running a program it called IWASH—Improved Water, Sanitation and Hygiene—in the three rural counties, with money from the U.S. Agency for International Development (USAID). The program was meant to halt unnecessary deaths caused by preventable diseases like cholera and typhoid, diseases caused by unsanitary drinking-water supplies.

The Global Communities teams that would show up in small rural villages were always made up of Liberians from nearby areas so they could demonstrate tribal ties. They hoped to spur behavior change by linking actions to health outcomes. If a latrine were situated near a water source, the teams told villagers, they were at risk for preventable disease. It was up to the community to take responsibility for their own water safety—a message that worked much better than one delivered by an outsider demanding an end to decades or centuries of local custom. The teams had to break the stigma of speaking openly about feces, and about the links between feces and illnesses like diarrhea.

In many villages, before Global Communities arrived, those links just didn't exist; villagers believed someone got sick because of a curse or because of occult magic.

The partnership between Global Communities and the local villages was forged by environmental health technicians. They were technically employed by county governmental health teams, though Global Communities helped fund the $80 per month they made as they zipped between villages on their motorcycles.

But after a decade, the work of Global Communities was nearing an end. In March 2014, deVries had held his first meeting with the Liberian Ministry of Health about wrapping up his group's involvement, and handing over control of the IWASH program to the government.

Days later, Ebola's presence was confirmed in Guinea, and the first cases were trickling over the border into Liberia. DeVries traveled north to Lofa County, where a health official told him to go to the town of Foya, on the border just south of the outbreak's epicenter. DeVries felt a fear he hadn't felt before. The atmosphere was scary, he said later.

Instead of handing over the IWASH program, deVries and his partner at Global Communities, Brett Sedgewick, debated another course of action: Global Communities was the only nongovernmental organization with a significant presence in the rural north. Its environmental health technicians were known to the village leaders on the front lines of the fight against Ebola. If the Liberian government or some other NGO couldn't deliver a credible message about the deadly virus because of deep-seated mistrust, maybe the well-regarded Global Communities teams could. The IWASH program became the Assisting Liberians with Education to Reduce Transmission—ALERT—program. USAID wrote the group another check, for a modest $760,000.[3]

The environmental health technicians, who had been used to traveling on bumpy rural roads to deliver messages about clean water, would be trained in something new: the safe burial and disposal of virus-infected bodies.

Across the border in Sierra Leone, David Robinson's network found itself in a similar position. Robinson worked for World Vision, the global charity best known in the United States for its advertisements seeking sponsors for children living in extreme poverty in desperately poor countries. The group had 58,000 children enrolled in its program in Sierra Leone, overseen by a staff of about 300 operating on a $12 million annual budget. Like Global Communities in Liberia, World Vision had a long relationship with communities in rural Sierra Leone; its staff had shown up during Sierra Leone's civil war, helping to disarm and reintegrate members of the rebel army back into society.

When Robinson, based in World Vision's regional capital in Dakar, Senegal, first visited Sierra Leone in May 2014, he found a country in denial, even as Ebola cases mounted. He facilitated a World Vision airlift of some of the first personal protection equipment into the country.

At first, Robinson saw World Vision as an important conduit to the thriving faith community in Sierra Leone. Schools and universities had been shuttered and markets went bare, but religious services continued. In many parts of the country, services at churches and mosques were the only places where large groups of people continued gathering. Before chlorine-based hand-washing stations became ubiquitous sights around the country, some of the first appeared in churches and mosques where World Vision had built a decade-long relationship.

Most important, as in Liberia, ministers and imams were trustworthy messengers, even as mistrust in government remained.

By September, the World Health Organization approached Robinson with a request that sounded similar to what they asked of deVries in Liberia: Could World Vision—along with Caritas, a Catholic charity based in the United Kingdom, and Islamic Relief—help rethink Sierra Leone's traditional burial practices, to cut down on transmissions between dead bodies and survivors?

World Vision had been hearing from religious leaders that their traditions had been overlooked, sowing still more distrust in the westerners who purported to help Sierra Leone's rural communities. WHO's approach to what it called "dead body management" sounded clinical, disrespectful.

Instead of letting their loved ones be carted away, unwashed, and dumped in a mass grave, villagers would hide bodies or refuse access to some of the early burial teams who showed up in protective equipment.

In smaller towns outside Freetown, faith leaders became the messengers who spread word of Ebola to a skeptical populace. In Bo, the regional capital in eastern Sierra Leone, Robinson watched as two particular preachers—a Christian pastor named Peter Kainwo and one Imam Koker—united their congregations in the fight. Kainwo and Koker visited each other's congregations to share messages about Ebola. Their mantra became: Doctrine divides, service unites.

Burial teams were already operating in other parts of Sierra Leone and Liberia, though few thought to implement them widely. In Monrovia, a city with a population of more than a million people, just six teams of body collectors were working by July 2014. Each team, clad head to toe in personal protective equipment, picked up at least half a dozen bodies a day. Some days, they collected twenty-five or more, delivering them to the crematorium set up outside the city. It was not uncommon for the teams in Monrovia to visit the same block of houses—or even the same home— multiple times, to collect the remains of friends, neighbors, and family members who had infected each other.

Even in cosmopolitan Monrovia, where messages about the danger of Ebola were omnipresent, denial ran rampant. Residents of the overcrowded slums routinely told burial teams that their family members had died from a miscarriage, or a stroke, or any of a hundred other maladies, when even the most basically trained health care provider could see that Ebola was almost certainly present.[4]

Out in the rural counties, burial teams encountered more resistance. Locals did not trust the government, run by the descendants of former American slaves, and centuries of tradition demanded that families take care of their own dead bodies. Muslim villages felt particularly strongly about caring for their own dead, especially if the members of a burial team were non-Muslim.

The Global Communities teams, however, found themselves in a unique position. They had forged relations over a decade with village elders throughout the three rural counties—and, along the way, they had shown results, as the number of deaths from cholera and other preventable diseases plummeted after the IWASH system took hold. Now those same teams were returning to the villages they knew so well, promising once again to end the scourge of disease. The environmental health technicians-turned burial teams paid special attention to cultural sensitivities: Muslim bodies were handled only by a specially created all-Muslim burial team.

Even having developed years of relationships, convincing villagers to give up sacred tradition proved difficult. In every community, the teams had to convince families and village elders that they were there for the right reasons.

"It convinced [village] leadership that what we were doing was a real health concern, and not some conspiracy by the government," deVries explained later.

In Sierra Leone, World Vision employed its own version of cultural finesse. Its program integrated burial teams and faith leaders. The burial teams, some trained in Christian traditions, others in Muslim traditions, would collect the bodies and bury them in marked graves, giving families a physical location at which to grieve and honor the deceased. At the same time, faith leaders were invited to be present at burials, to offer prayers and counseling.

It was a new mission for an old organization, one that World Vision had to learn on the fly.

"No NGO is known to have a specialty as an undertaker. Working with burial teams is not something we would list as an organizational specialty. Nobody does," Robinson said.

Having been dispatched to pick up a body, burial team leaders would make their first stop at the home of the deceased. They would speak with the family and with community leaders to explain step by step what they had arrived to do. As was custom, the burial teams—handpicked to come from nearby villages—would explain their tribal ties to the village, to prove they shared common foundations. They asked to hear about the life of the deceased; often, families would deny their relative had even fallen ill. Denial was easier than acceptance of an invisible microbe in their midst.

Soon after the IWASH teams had become Ebola-fighting burial teams, deVries accompanied his men to a village where a suspected victim lay. After what seemed like hours of talk between the team and the dead man's family, as they established a careful rapport, a village elder stepped forward to say there had been other strange deaths, after a visitor from Monrovia arrived. The elder's wife had died, then another friend, and now this man. The villagers realized Ebola was among them.

The family led the burial team, six Liberians from nearby villages, to the body, down a hill, through a swampy marsh, across a rickety bridge that was little more than wooden branches strung together with twine. They came to an island in the marsh, where crops were growing around the body.

Together, the burial team suited up in full-body protective equipment, under the blazing equatorial sun. One member of the team sprayed chlorine on every available surface, to kill any virus lurking about. They hoisted the dead body, oozing with blood, onto their shoulders and retraced their steps, through knee-deep marsh water and up the steep hill to a waiting grave, dug by the man's family. As the burial team explained every step to villagers, they lowered the body into the grave and filled it with dirt. Villagers attended the burial, though they were kept well back.

It was not long before Global Communities' work started to show some promise. Case counts in Monrovia continued to rise, but the rates of new infections in Bong, Lofa, and Nimba Counties began to tail off. Through August and September, just as the American response began to ramp up, USAID took notice. Soon, deVries got a phone call from a senior USAID officer: How soon, the officer asked, could you set up burial teams in other counties?

Within weeks, Global Communities teams were everywhere in northern counties, overseen by a tall, commanding Liberian named George Woryonwon. Dubbed Uncle George by the environmental health technicians he had managed for years, he was known as a fixer. When one of the burial teams had a problem with a motorcycle, or when their salaries didn't arrive in time, or when they needed some vital equipment, they called Uncle George. He came through.

Now he burned up the phone lines, establishing burial teams through as many county health offices as he could reach. Once those burial teams were set up, Global Communities would ship in the personal protective equipment, the body bags, vehicles, and supplies. Each team got three vehicles: an ambulance to carry the body, a truck to carry the burial team, and a second truck to carry those who would spray an affected area thoroughly with chlorine. In Monrovia, deVries was buying as many cars and trucks as he could get his hands on.

"We had every jalopy that was available in very rural places," he said.

The remoteness of rural West Africa is difficult to comprehend. Communities can be an hour's walk from the nearest passable road. The Liberian burial teams carried supplies on their heads, through thick jungle along barely visible trails. Some burial teams took canoes through murky rivers, which meant they needed life preservers. After retrieving a body, oarsmen would paddle canoes back downstream, still clad in full protective gear.

In Sierra Leone, where World Vision worked in some larger cities, they took extreme precautions to protect their employees. Staff were not allowed to attend burials, and they were not allowed to eat outside the office. World Vision satellite offices built their own kitchens to feed staffers.

By September, the first Global Communities–backed burial teams arrived in southeastern and northwestern Liberian counties, areas where the group had not operated before. It was the middle of the rainy season, and roads turned so bad that what should have been a long day's drive turned into a several-night-long odyssey.

While the international response had focused on Monrovia and the rural northern counties, the virus had moved south and east, decimating new counties that had gone overlooked. Parts of those counties remained out of government reach even after cessation of Liberia's civil war; now they felt neglected. The communications efforts that had so rapidly raised awareness in the capital and even up north had not reached the southeast. The problems with a parallel governing structure that had vexed some Ebola response efforts in Bong, Lofa, and Nimba Counties were doubly difficult in the southeast, where tribal governance dominated and Monrovia's control was symbolic, at best.

The first Global Communities burial teams met resistance, some of it violent. In River Cess County, south of Nimba along the Atlantic coast, a mob commandeered one burial team's vehicles. The team had to walk home. To the east, in Sinoe County, a mob stoned the house where a new burial team was being trained.

In Monrovia, a group of traditional elders, led by the paramount chief, Zanzan Kawa, came to see deVries at Global Communities headquarters. They offered to help in any way they could, and deVries thanked them for coming. Still, he could not immediately think of a way they might be of service—and he did not immediately grasp the significance of the role they played. After he escorted the elders to the door, one of his Liberian staff members pulled him aside: That was the National Traditional Leadership Council, the staffer explained. It was the equivalent to the traditional government what a president's cabinet is to a formal government. They needed those leaders on their side if Global Communities was going to have any chance of introducing itself to communities in the southeast.

DeVries called Kawa back to ask for help. They would need to break down the barriers between traditional government and the federal government, they agreed, to coordinate supplies and help to these new communities just now being introduced to Ebola. The National Traditional Leadership Council helped set up partnerships with local county health offices. The tribal leaders would introduce the health-care workers to village elders, giving them an important endorsement as the health-care workers brought with them the foreign concept of burial teams.

So Global Communities started over. Led by another veteran of the IWASH program, Tamba Boima, the group and its partners from the council and county health offices held community meetings across River Cess and Sinoe Counties to introduce Ebola, to give a name to the deadly virus stalking their villages, and to lay the groundwork for burial teams. Between August and December, Boima and his colleagues met with more than 15,000 community leaders in the two counties.

Soon, the first ambulances arrived, as Boima had promised. Community leaders got the message: the capital cared about them, and help was on the way. Traditional leaders asked their fellow tribesmen to end bush schools, those secret societies that performed rituals like circumcision—potent havens for transmission.

Back in Monrovia, another Global Communities staffer was having trouble with the outbreak. Before Ebola, Freeman Kamara, the group's Liberian accountant, was used to a desk job, where he kept the books and made sure the environmental health technicians got paid. But once the outbreak began, and especially after USAID asked Global Communities to expand its burial team practice so rapidly, he was pressed into a different kind of service.

There are few working ATMs in Liberia. Outside Monrovia, there are hardly any. While the Western world has moved on to credit cards and electronic payments, West Africa still runs on cash. Someone had to pay the hundreds of new employees on the Global Communities payroll, and that job often fell to Kamara. He was frequently dispatched from the safety of his desk to the rural, remote roads in a jeep laden with $50,000 or $100,000 in cash, money stuffed into backpacks or hidden in secret compartments in the floor.

Because of the remoteness of the burial teams who worked for Global Communities, Kamara often found himself on long walks through the jungle, or on canoe trips up long rivers. He couldn't swim; after deVries posted a photo of Kamara on the group's Facebook page describing their often-treacherous treks, Global Communities was inundated by offers to send Freeman a life jacket.

As the rainy season ended, public health officials in Washington and Geneva watched as the instances of postmortem transmission in rural counties where burial teams were operating plateaued, and then tailed off. It was hard to escape the conclusion that a solution—not a silver bullet, but a long-term solution—was at hand. A total of twenty-seven Global Communities–run ambulances ended up stationed in key sectors around Liberia.

"The number one driver of transmission reduction were the burial teams," said Rajiv Shah, who headed USAID during the outbreak. "The Global Communities people single-handedly did more to solve Ebola in Liberia than any other partner on the planet, including all the doctors put together."

"They understood how to go into those communities without terrifying people and being generally respectful at a community burial, which, you know, had very ingrained social practices that you're trying to change in a rapid form," Shah said. There were times when ambulances funded by USAID and run by Global Communities burial teams showed up near villages before Ebola did.

But in Washington, one of Shah's closest advisers, Jeremy Konyndyk, was puzzling over some troubling data. Health officials led by the British military were operating burial teams in Sierra Leone, with only a fraction of the success they found in Liberia. In Liberia, burial teams arrived at a home to find an Ebola victim untouched; in Sierra Leone, they often found bodies lying serenely on a bed, washed, cleaned, and dressed—which negated the point of burial teams meant to limit contact between the deceased and those who could become the virus's next generation of victims.

Health officials came up with two main theories for the discrepancy. On one hand, those who set up burial teams in Liberia were well-known to and trusted by a local community. Aside from World Vision, those who set up burial teams in Sierra Leone and later in Guinea were usually the military or foreign organizations, both groups that generated their share of skepticism in villages where burial teams were most urgently needed. The second theory was that most rural villages in Sierra Leone were Muslim communities, where religious tradition demanded a stricter set of burial practices.

While Freeman Kamara bounced and bumped his way along rural roads to pay Global Communities workers, emergency health professionals in other parts of West Africa were not being paid. On November 25, a burial team based at the hospital in Kenema, Sierra Leone, dumped three bodies— two adults and a child, all victims of Ebola—in front of the hospital's gates, to protest the lack of pay. The twenty-three members of the burial team were owed €100 a week, or about $115, in hazard pay. They had seen no money for two months. (After the entire team was fired, some members continued working for tips.)[5]

The problem of unpaid workers extended far beyond Kenema, more evidence of a woefully inadequate health-care system in a nation rife with corruption. Before the central government could issue payments, it had to build a list of its actual employees. When the World Bank stepped in to ensure that hazard payments would get to emergency workers, they found corruption on a massive scale. Some Ministry of Health officials had created dozens of false names to which paychecks were being issued. Others had put relatives on the employment rolls for no-show jobs and pocketed their pay.

As late as November, the government was handing out cash to its employees. By December, they had set up a direct deposit system, managed by a small team representing the United Nations Development Programme based in Freetown, either to bank accounts or to cell phone accounts, in a country where many people still did not use Western banking systems. Officials from the UN had to sign off on payrolls before anyone got a check, to stem corruption. Soon, 23,000 nurses were paid a total of €21 million through the system.

By the end of the year, about $3.3 billion in donations had been sent to West Africa to fight Ebola, and more than one hundred nongovernmental organizations were helping in various capacities. But little of that money went to those who put their lives on the line. Nurses in the Kenema hospital were paid just €80 a week, or about $92. Some had second jobs. Others charged patients under the table for extra care, to supplement their meager incomes.

Medical personnel in Sierra Leone treating Ebola patients directly received €100 a week, the same as burial teams, in hazard pay. Nurses in general wards got an extra €40 for their trouble. Even as health officials arrived from Britain and the United States, Kenema's hospital still lacked the most basic medical supplies; one doctor from the United States began fashioning medical aprons out of tarpaulins.[6]

Around all three countries, Ebola treatment units continued opening at a rapid pace. The first facility built by the U.S. military opened on November 18 in Tubmanburg, in Bomi County, west of Monrovia. Three more Army-built facilities opened around Liberia in December. Médecins Sans Frontières opened a laboratory and an emergency management center in Freetown, at the Prince of Wales School, on December 10.

When a new outbreak sprang up in Gbarpolu County, along the border with Sierra Leone, Global Communities once again sent burial teams to squelch it. Though it is only a few dozen miles as the crow flies from Tubmanburg and Monrovia, Gbarpolu County redefines the concept of remoteness; Global Communities had to virtually rent out the only canoe ferry across the Mano River to gain access to the affected villages.

Back in Monrovia, a reversal of fortune had taken place. For decades, it had been the rural communities that harbored resentments toward the governing elite, the descendants of American slaves holed up in the capital who ran a government that favored residents of Monrovia over tribal communities elsewhere. But since August 5, when President Ellen Johnson Sirleaf had ordered bodies in the capital cremated to reduce the risk of Ebola transmissions, it had been those in Monrovia who felt their countrymen in the bush were getting the better deal. Cremation was so foreign to the Liberian concept of death and dying; at least the burial teams up north were washing the deceased and giving them a proper resting place.

Just as traditional tribal leaders became so important in the bush, where they convinced villagers to welcome the burial teams, traditional leaders in Monrovia began taking on a more important role. Cremations had never sat well with Zanzan Kawa, the paramount chief. Sirleaf had mandated cremation not for any nefarious reason; the Ministry of Health was simply running out of places to put dead bodies. Now Kawa appealed to fellow members of the National Traditional Leadership Council to help find a new site for a massive cemetery, one that would give Ebola victims a proper burial, and a proper entrée into the afterlife.

Tribes from around Monrovia offered as many options as they could. Officials from the Ministry of Health, the Ministry of Internal Affairs and the Ministry of Lands, Mines and Energy surveyed each successive site. They examined whether it had enough space, whether it was high enough above the water table to survive the long rainy season, and whether it was accessible to ambulances that would bring in the dead.

By October, they had found a site, one offered by Chief Kawa's own tribe. The plot of land was called Disco Hill, where a western company used to harvest rubber east of Monrovia in Margibi County. Once the tribe could formally transfer ownership of the land, Global Communities, thanks to a grant from USAID's Office of Foreign Development Assistance (OFDA), would be able to hire the workers necessary to transform an overgrown forest into a dignified resting place.

But in a country where nothing seems easy, transferring land presented more unexpected hurdles. Land titles had been the source of contention and distrust between the governing elite and tribes since the former African American slaves first landed in what is now Monrovia. And while Chief Kawa's tribe offered the land for sale for just $50,000—an amount that represented more of a token payment than a serious transaction—the Ministry of Internal Affairs prohibited the sale. Money from the OFDA, a foreign government agency, could not be used to buy Liberian land.

The delay particularly bothered Tolbert Nyenswah. Nyenswah had been driven from his home in 1993, during the beginning of the civil war, when he was forced to spend years in a migrant camp in Côte d'Ivoire. He had returned home after receiving a law degree and a master's in public health from Johns Hopkins University. When Ebola broke out, Nyenswah had been dispatched from his job as Liberia's deputy minister of health to become head of the Incident Management System, the agency overseeing Liberia's response to the outbreak. He told friends he couldn't believe that such an important step, necessary to stop the cremations that threatened to sow more discord in Monrovia, had been blocked by a government bureaucrat.

After days of torturous back and forth, the Ministry of Internal Affairs decided they would simply buy the land themselves. Workers were already clearing forest and leveling territory; within days, they had created a burial area for Christian victims of Ebola, and one for Muslim victims.

But the ministry's check had not arrived, and no check meant no bodies. Several times, the landowners had to tell the teams to stop work until the check came through. And while some Liberian customs flummoxed western aid workers, bureaucratic slowdowns and screwups were the same the world over. One check arrived, but it was made out to the wrong person. Another check showed up days later, but for only half the amount necessary to transfer the land.

In December, two months after Chief Kawa's tribe had identified the site on Disco Hill, Senator Chris Coons arrived in Liberia. The former missionary was the first American elected official to set foot in West Africa during the outbreak, and he had been following the controversy over the cemetery. He brought it up in a meeting with Sirleaf: Why hadn't this simple act, this cutting of a check, been taken care of? Sirleaf promised to find out.

Two days later, on December 23, the check—made out to the right recipient, for the right amount—was signed. Sirleaf issued a declaration formally ending the national policy that all dead bodies must be cremated that same day. On December 24, the first Ebola victim was buried at Disco Hill.

For the next several months, the dead found a resting place at the cemetery, albeit one that was far more regimented than a normal burial site. Burial teams similar to those who roamed the northern counties met every arriving ambulance. Every body bag, every grave was completely sprayed down by a disinfection team, dressed in full protective gear, wearing backpacks equipped with chlorine sprayers. The entire facility was separated by orange plastic fences, demarcating red zones where Ebola might be present, and blue zones where protective gear was not required.

From an ambulance, a body would be carried to a temporary morgue. Three identification cards traveled with the body at all times, to ensure that families knew where their loved ones rested. Grave-diggers, who worked in teams of four, could excavate a final resting place in about five hours; once a location was ready, the six members of the burial team would lower the deceased, body bag and all, carefully into the ground. The chlorine sprayer stayed behind to disinfect everything that might have come into contact with the body.

A year after the Disco Hill cemetery opened, Global Communities formally transferred control of the site to the Liberian Ministry of Health. On January 19, 2015, Matt Ward, the group's site director, handed an oversized key to a Ministry of Health official in an elaborate ceremony. Three thousand Ebola victims rested beneath their feet. The ashes of thousands more who had been cremated between August 5 and December 23, transferred to a newly built mausoleum, had found their resting place, too.

In Sierra Leone, not one of the 58,000 sponsored children involved in World Vision's programs contracted the Ebola virus.

EIGHTEEN

A Waning Tide

WHEN LEISHA NOLEN RETURNED to Sierra Leone in November, she felt as if she were visiting a different country from the one she left in August. After her last deployment, the normally active Centers for Disease Control and Prevention (CDC) Epidemic Intelligence Service officer had been so depressed about the spiraling virus that she sat, moribund, on her couch for weeks on end. During that deployment, the daily case counts were growing by the dozens—on some days, by the hundreds. Nolen and some of her colleagues spent their time in Sierra Leone and Liberia wondering whether they, or anyone, could actually get a handle on the growing crisis. The looks on the faces of the Sierra Leoneans she worked with were grim; unlike Nolen, they were not going to rotate home for a break. Their home was the one on fire.

But a few months later, Nolen found a different situation entirely. Her third deployment took her to Kambia, in northern Sierra Leone, a town of about 40,000 inhabitants about halfway between Freetown and Conakry. The number of reported, suspected, and probable cases of Ebola in West Africa continued to rise, from about 4,800 at the beginning of November to 7,100 by the beginning of December, but Nolen detected a notable change in the country's mood.

Employees working for the CDC, Médecins Sans Frontières (MSF), Global Communities, and others detected the same change in the last few months of the year. The case curve, which just a few months before had been growing exponentially, was starting to level off. Elders in villages facing the virus for the first time were no longer skeptical that Ebola existed; instead, they started asking questions about how to stop the spread of the danger in their midst, a credit to the national education programs airing on radio stations around all three countries. The international response had finally caught up with the severity of the outbreak, to the extent that even smaller countries were contributing what they could. The Dutch government spent more than €18,000 for a Stop Ebola card game, modeled on the game Memory.[1]

In his morning meetings, Major General Gary Volesky began to see a downward trend in new case counts. Every day, Volesky would review the "heartbeat chart," a graph that showed weeklong averages of new cases and projections of cases in the future, which gave responders a sense of which regions needed urgent attention. The upward curve that resembled a hockey stick when he arrived had begun to bend slowly downward through November.

"By December, you're saying, wow, there's less than 30 cases reported total a day," Volesky said. But he remained leery: A single person had started the initial outbreak in Guinea. A single person had spread the virus over the border into Liberia. A single person had brought Ebola to the heart of Monrovia, sparking an outbreak in densely packed urban slums. "It only took one person to start this before," he said later.

A new cluster of Ebola cases in Cape Mount County, on Liberia's northern border with Sierra Leone, showed just how much progress the nation had made. Even before the first cases popped up, burial teams trained by Global Communities were patrolling villages in Cape Mount. The first bodies those teams were called to pick up showed that the villagers still did not fully buy into the virus's lethality—the bodies had been washed and dressed for the afterlife.

But where education efforts directed by Monrovia's government had not worked, the nongovernmental organizations (NGOs) working in Cape Mount turned to their second line of attack: traditional leaders.

Cape Mount is a predominantly Muslim county, one of the few in Liberia. So Global Communities found the highest-ranking Muslim traditional leader they could: Musa Kamara, who headed the Paramount Chiefs Council, a group of traditional elders, in neighboring Lofa County. Chief Kamara had seen the toll Ebola took on villages in his Quardu Gboni District, and he knew how urgent it was for Cape Mount to take action quickly. A day after receiving a call asking him to visit, he was in the car.

Once he arrived, Chief Kamara and a local grand mufti organized a meeting with traditional leaders in Cape Mount, especially those who were skeptical about the virus. The disease is real, they told their counterparts. After the meeting broke up, the chief visited nearby villages to spread his message beyond the traditional leadership. Ebola, Kamara said, was survivable, but only if those who were ill sought treatment in time. Save Cape Mount, he urged villagers, from the horror Lofa went through.

Within days, those who had fallen ill started showing up at newly built Ebola treatment units. Where the government in Monrovia had little credibility, Kamara had served as an important validator of the point they were trying to get across. The mistrust between traditional leaders and the central government might still exist, but the two sides knew when they needed to work together.

As the infection curve bent downward and as virus hunters started believing they could strangle the disease, a new batch of scientists began arriving, a group more accustomed to dealing with the microscopic, rather than the human, element of an outbreak.

Just as virus hunters had arrived in West Africa sensing the opportunity of a lifetime, their best chance to practice their craft under the highest possible pressure, so too did microbiologists see an opportunity in the Ebola outbreak.

Before 2014, only a relatively small number of people had ever come into contact with the Zaire strain of the virus, dubbed EBOV—and even fewer had caught any of the three relatives that have been shown to harm humans. Only 1,383 known cases of the EBOV, or Zaire, strain had been diagnosed before the outbreak in West Africa; just 778 cases of the Sudan strain (SUDV) had been diagnosed. Over the course of just two known outbreaks, 185 people had come down with the Bundibugyo (BDBV) strain. And the Tai Forest virus had been found only a single time in that one unfortunate Swiss graduate student, working in the nature preserve in Côte d'Ivoire in 1994.[2] In almost every outbreak, the Ebola virus burned through a population so fast that the disease had disappeared before microbiologists arrived to study it.

Put another way, before the outbreak in West Africa, scientists knew little about one of the scariest viruses on the planet—which meant that their efforts to create new treatments and vaccines had not progressed as fast as with other, better understood diseases. Lab tests at places like the U.S. Army Medical Research Institute for Infectious Diseases (USAMRIID) and the CDC could only go so far. Seeing the virus in the wild, understanding how it morphed and mutated between patients, would give scientists an invaluable leg up in the war against such a deadly pathogen.

Captain Jeff Kugelman was among the first genetics experts deployed to Liberia to slice open Ebola virions in hopes of finding new ways to prevent the next wave of infections. Trained as a viral geneticist at the University of Texas at El Paso, Kugelman, bespectacled and with the shaved head of a career Army man, is serious about his work at USAMRIID. He arrived in Monrovia on November 17, 2014, armed with an Illumina MiSeq, a high-tech gene sequencer about the size of an office printer.

The MiSeq is an extremely expensive, extremely delicate machine, designed to sequence the genetics of any given specimen. Sequencing any Ebola virion, isolating the base pairs of A, T, C, and G proteins that make up RNA, would take between three and seven days; Kugelman's mission was to sequence as many samples as possible, to understand the various threads of infection that had radiated out from Meliandou nearly a year beforehand. Diagramming those infection chains would help virologists understand how Ebola spread, and how it had mutated along the way.

The company that produced the machine knew it would not be able to send engineers to the hot zone to conduct repairs in case something went wrong, so Kugelman took a two-week course to become a certified engineer qualified to fix the MiSeq. Illumina bent over backward to help, maintaining a twenty-four-hour rotation of technicians based in London and the United States to advise Kugelman if he needed help. The technicians and the course came in handy immediately. The day Kugelman ar-

rived, the local contractor hauling the sequencer to his makeshift laboratory dropped the box. The machine broke, but Kugelman had the skills to
repair it using only the tools at his disposal.

"It survived a pretty close to worst-case scenario," Kugelman chuckled
later, nervously eyeing his delicate machine as it sat on his desk at Fort
Detrick.

Kugelman set up shop near Liberia's airport, at the Monrovia Medical
Unit, the Ebola treatment unit that had been reserved for any Westerners
who might come down with the virus. The facility was designed as a crude
horseshoe, built of cinderblocks, with nothing more than a covered breeze-
way connecting his lab to the treatment unit. It had been a forward staging
base for the U.S. Navy during World War II, and so it had a few apartments, though Kugelman stayed closer to town at an Army hotel, an hour
down the road.

From the start, Kugelman and his small team had to cart in virtually
everything they needed to do their work. Their lab had no clean water, no
fuel for generators that kept the machines whirring. They were working
on a biosafety level-4 (BSL-4) pathogen in what amounted to BSL-2 conditions, with far fewer safety precautions than they might have liked. Kugelman kept three backup battery packs, each with about seven hours of
life, on standby to make sure the MiSeq and their computers would not
shut off in the middle of hours-long sequencing processes, so they
wouldn't lose their work. Power spikes kept blowing out converters as
surges coursed through the system. The results they generated would
lead to a better understanding of how Ebola worked—and later, the virus's lasting effects on someone who had survived its initial, devastating
onslaught.

As Kugelman worked, the first Army-built Ebola treatment units began
opening in Liberia. But by then, the infection curve had begun to level
off from its exponential growth in September, October, and the early part
of November. That meant the demand for beds to treat Ebola patients
dropped, and the Army had to decide whether to continue building the
facilities already under construction. It was becoming clear that the military had planned to build more facilities than would actually be needed—a
conundrum that led to some criticism back home, but Army officials

thought it was a better problem than the one they would have faced had they built fewer than the number of facilities required.[3]

The initial plans had called for as many as 30 new American-built Ebola treatment units across Liberia, expanding treatment capacity by 3,000 beds. Even knowing many of those beds would never be occupied by an Ebola patient, the Pentagon, in consultation with the White House, decided to finish the units already under construction. At the very least, they would serve as new medical facilities Liberia could use to begin rebuilding a health-care system already decimated by the virus. In the worst-case scenario, if Ebola had staged yet another comeback, the facilities would be ready to receive a new wave of patients.

"We couldn't really be confident until December or January, when it was really clear that cases really were turning down and we had turned a corner in a pretty significant way in Liberia. We couldn't be certain that we wouldn't eventually need" all thirty planned facilities, Jeremy Konyndyk of the United States Agency for International Development (USAID) Office of Foreign Disaster Assistance said. "It's much, much worse to get it wrong and try to catch up than to overdo it a little bit to be on the safe side."

Still, even with the curve bending down, new facilities opened up at a breakneck pace. After months of inaction, and setbacks driven by fears surrounding the infections of Kent Brantly and Nancy Writebol, the global community was now more engaged than ever in the responses. Germany's government funded new Ebola treatment units, even after there weren't enough patients to fill beds. So did the Chinese government. Nongovernmental organizations that had stayed away in early months now built their own facilities.

Hans Rosling and Luke Bawo realized what had happened. Now that some NGOs had demonstrated their effectiveness, everyone else was rushing in to claim some kind of credit. Every NGO wanted to show its donors that they had helped, and to show news media broadcasting on channels watched by European and American donors that they were in the game. The Liberian Ministry of Health gamely let several NGOs hold elaborate opening ceremonies for the cameras, then quietly closed the facilities or reappropriated them for more pressing medical needs.

"The world was generous," Rosling said. "To coordinate [all the new facilities], that was the difficulty."

Back in Washington, the approaching holidays presented the White House's Ebola response team with its most critical challenge. Ron Klain's strategy, from the day he returned to the White House to oversee the fight against the virus, had been to keep careful tabs on visitors and citizens entering the country from Liberia, Sierra Leone, and Guinea. On a typical day, that meant monitoring between 1,300 and 1,400 people, a manageable task. But with Christmas just around the corner, that number ballooned to 2,700 people traveling from West Africa.

Public health departments were already stretched thin. Many staffers took vacation over the holidays, and the health departments wanted to know: Would travelers have to continue checking in to report their temperatures and any outward signs of illness on Christmas Day? Yes, Klain decided, they absolutely had to check in.

Klain had spent most of his weeks as Ebola czar cocooned inside the White House, or shuttling between USAID and Secretary Sylvia Burwell's office at the Department of Health and Human Services. But a week before Christmas, he got his first chance to come face to face with a group of Americans who had gone overseas to fight the outbreak. The Americans who returned were young volunteers from the U.S. Public Health Service (PHS), doctors and nurses who traded their service for help in paying their student bills. Under ordinary circumstances, the Public Health Service members were deployed to Native American reservations and other communities that struggled to maintain adequate modern health services. These volunteers had been dispatched to care for Ebola patients at the Monrovia Medical Unit where Kugelman had been based.

After these volunteers arrived back in the United States, some of the communities the Public Health Service served were wary about their returning before the twenty-one-day quarantine period ended. The Public Health Service did not require its employees to quarantine themselves, but those who wanted or needed to stay away were put up in a Holiday Inn in Gaithersburg, up the road from Washington along Interstate 270.

The idea of a bunch of public servants spending the holidays alone and far from home did not sit well with Klain. "They had gone to West Africa, they had fought this disease. They weren't allowed to go home," he remembered later.

So the White House invited them for a visit, the day after Christmas, while Obama was in Hawaii on his annual winter vacation. Klain's team showed the young doctors the West Wing, led them on a tour of the rest of the White House, and let them bowl in the president's bowling alley. Klain brought his family, too. None of the PHS workers ever came down with the virus.

As the new year began, the slowing rate of Ebola cases illustrated the number of communities that had gotten the epidemic under control. On January 27, Médecins Sans Frontières closed its Ebola management center (EMC) in Kailahun, Sierra Leone, after forty-two days—two incubation periods—without a new case. Around the same time, the EMC in Bo discharged its last confirmed patients. MSF staff redeployed to Freetown, where they opened a new treatment center to help the capital end its outbreak. The last Army-built Ebola treatment centers opened in Liberia on January 28; of the eleven treatment units that the Army built, nine never treated a single patient.

The Army was stricter with returning service members than the PHS had been. When Tony Costello arrived home in Texas, he was quarantined at an old National Guard training center at North Fort Hood for twenty-one days, even though he had never even seen a patient afflicted with the Ebola virus. He thought the quarantine was overkill, but he spent his time honing his video game skills with fellow officers.

As the military began rotating troops home, and once the federal government had helped local hospitals develop their own domestic Ebola treatment capabilities, Klain began to feel that his work was done. He had been called in to create a wholly new capability to treat a deadly disease, and now it was time to fold that capability back into the normal structure of government. When Klain arrived at the White House, laboratory facilities in just thirteen states had the technical ability to test for the Ebola virus, and only three hospitals were capable of treating an Ebola patient. By the time he left, fifty-four labs in forty-four states could run those tests, and fifty-one medical facilities were capable of treating an Ebola patient.

"We could tell the epidemic was nearing an end in West Africa, the U.S. response was up and working well, and it seemed like it was time to turn off an extraordinary response and put it back into the system," Klain said. By early February, he was packing up, preparing to return to his day job working for Steve Case.

But before Klain left, he helped to stage-manage some public recognition for the work that Americans from a dizzying array of backgrounds had done to stem the outbreak. On February 11, four days before Klain's last day on the job, President Obama stood before dozens of employees and volunteers from the CDC, USAMRIID, USAID, and the National Institutes of Health, along with a handful of NGOs, to thank them, and to highlight just what they had done. In remarks carried live by several cable news networks Obama said:

Last summer, as Ebola spread in West Africa, overwhelming public health systems and threatening to cross more borders, I said that fighting this disease had to be more than a national security priority, but an example of American leadership. After all, whenever and wherever a disaster or a disease strikes, the world looks to us to lead. And because of extraordinary people like the ones standing behind me, and many who are in the audience, we have risen to the challenge. . . . People were understandably afraid, and, if we're honest, some stoked those fears. But we believed that if we made policy based not on fear, but on sound science and good judgment, America could lead an effective global response while keeping the American people safe, and we could turn the tide of the epidemic.

By the end of April, Obama said, all but one hundred of the thousands of Americans dispatched to West Africa would be home. But the job, Obama stressed, was not over.

"Our focus now is getting to zero [cases]. Because as long as there is even one case of Ebola that's active out there, risks still exist. Every case is an ember that, if not contained, can light a new fire. So we're shifting our focus from fighting the epidemic to now extinguishing it."[4]

Before he entered the South Court Auditorium to thank the responders, Obama had met some of the survivors of the disease. Brantly, Craig Spencer, Amber Vinson, Nina Pham, and a few others were there, along with their families. White House photographer Pete Souza snapped dozens of photos of the survivors hugging the president of the United States, a preplanned effort to remove the stigma of having served in West Africa.

After the event, Klain's team took the survivors back to a conference room at the Old Executive Office Building, the room where he had spent so many hours building foreign and domestic threat matrixes to get a handle on the growing outbreak. For what seemed like hours, they just sat and talked, sharing stories of the highest highs and the lowest lows they had experienced. Amber Vinson's mother said her family had to move; even months later, the local pizza shop would not deliver to her house. Someone kept leaving nasty messages on her doorstep.

Klain and Gayle Smith were struck by the extraordinary diversity in the room. Brantly, the deeply religious, deeply conservative doctor who worked for Franklin Graham, had shared an experience with Spencer, the liberal New York do-gooder bent on saving the world. Vinson is African American. Pham is Asian American. Writebol and her husband were much older than most of the others. Together, they represented a cross-section of what could be a divided country, brought together by their determination to help others and to do what was right.

If that sentiment was not enough to choke up even the most hardened political operative like Klain, Brantly pushed him over the edge.

"I went to Liberia because I was called by God," Brantly told the hushed room. "I became deathly ill. I was alone, I couldn't touch my children or my wife. I was going to die. And my government came to get me and saved my life."

One by one, tears began streaming down faces around the room.

NINETEEN

Medicine without Borders

AS THE CALENDAR CHANGED from 2014 to 2015, the World Health Organization's (WHO) weekly case count report showed the number of new Ebola cases in Guinea, Sierra Leone, and Liberia plunging, almost as quickly as the curve had risen in August, September and October.

In December, the three nations reported 3,272 new cases. In January, 1,886 people were infected; in February, 1,637 new cases; in March, 1,484; and just 1,120 in April. After months at the brink of a global catastrophe, the Ebola outbreak was coming under control.

As the number of new infections fell, scientists and public health officials faced new questions about those who had survived the disease, and new opportunities to unlock the secrets of the virus to prevent the next big outbreak.

Never before had so many people survived the Ebola virus. By official counts, more than 17,000 people had recovered from the disease. Thousands more survivors who never reported their symptoms probably meant that number was far higher. Ebola is unlike most other viruses, both in its contagiousness and its lethality. But it also leaves behind scars, mental and psychological, that few had anticipated.

Once someone recovers from Ebola, they cannot contract the virus again—which makes the antibodies in their blood so useful for transfusions.

But those survivors reported horrible nightmares and memory loss. More than half had serious muscle and joint problems. Three in five suffered eye problems, even blindness, according to a report compiled by Liberian epidemiologist Mosoka Fallah.[1] A team of WHO researchers who interacted with Ebola survivors beginning in the fall of 2014 began referring to what they called post-Ebola syndrome. It gave a name to the vacant stare in the eyes of the woman who had lost her husband who Tom Frieden had seen at the ELWA hospital in August 2014. Now thousands more people experienced those same symptoms.

A series of joint studies conducted by the National Institutes of Health, the Liberian Ministry of Health, and a handful of other medical institutes, based in Fallah's offices at John F. Kennedy Medical Center in Monrovia, revealed many of the most persistent symptoms. The Partnership for Research on Ebola Vaccines in Liberia, or PREVAIL, hoped to enroll 1,500 survivors of the viruses, and 6,000 of their closest contacts, for five years of studies.

The pervasive eye problems proved especially disturbing. Ian Crozier, an American physician who had come down with the virus in Sierra Leone in October, went back to his doctors after just two months, when his eye changed color. Those doctors drew samples through a needle from his eye, where they found a heavier viral load than had been in his blood weeks before.

The virus lived on, too, in semen. WHO had warned survivors to practice safe sex for ninety days after recovering, a period defined by a 1995 outbreak in Zaire when the virus was still evident nearly three months after recovery.

But in West Africa, some former patients still had Ebola present in their semen six, nine, and twelve months after they had been given a supposedly clean bill of health. A handful of flare-ups of the Ebola disease, from March to November 2015, started after survivors returned home and had intercourse with their spouses or partners. The PREVAIL studies found that more than a third of male survivors had the disease present in their semen at least once.[2] One survivor still had Ebola present eighteen months after he first showed symptoms.

Other studies showed just how deeply damaging the Ebola outbreak had been in all three countries, and how long the damage would linger. So many health-care workers had fallen ill, and so many had died, that even standard health-care practices had all but stopped. At the height of the outbreak, few hospitals conducted Caesarian sections on pregnant women. Malaria vaccinations ceased. Tuberculosis patients went untreated.

In all three nations, the toll was immense. Ebola had been disproportionately likely to hit those between the ages of fifteen and forty-four. Women were more likely than men to contract the disease, largely because of the cultural roles women played in caring for family members and funerary traditions. That meant those who were most likely to have been struck down by Ebola were the most able-bodied workers in society, and women in their prime childbearing years. Their losses were tragic not only for their families but for their nations. All three countries were left with a missing generation, one that cannot reach its full economic potential or raise the next generation of West African children.

Even before the virus broke out, health systems in West Africa had been among the poorest in the world. With the threat of Ebola lurking, those systems virtually shut down and patients stayed away from medical facilities, causing a cascade of otherwise preventable deaths from other, usually more manageable maladies. In Liberia, outpatient doctor visits had declined 61 percent. Vaccinations dropped by half, and measles broke out in Liberia and Guinea during the early months of 2015. HIV patients, tuberculosis patients, and malaria victims went without medicine.

"More people died because of Ebola than from Ebola," Tom Frieden said later. "It collapsed the health care systems."

Efforts to halt the spread of the virus by limiting public interactions came with their own negative downsides. After schools were closed in July 2014, the number of adolescent pregnancies skyrocketed. So did infant mortality rates. Violence against women and girls jumped dramatically.[3] The schools did not begin opening again until February and March of 2015. As many as 23,000 children lost one of their parents, or both.

As the crisis waned, the response effort mounted by Liberians, Sierra Leoneans, Guineans, and their international partners turned from containment to recovery. But the road to recovery would be—and still is—long. The global donor community had generously pledged more than $5 billion to help all three nations recover. But as is so often the case in humanitarian crises, those pledges did not always come through. By early 2016, more than a third of the money pledged by international donor nations, $1.9 billion, had not arrived to help, according to an Oxfam report. Oxfam said it couldn't even be certain that the remaining $3.9 billion pledged had arrived because donor nations do not always disclose what they give, and how.[4]

To help repair the damage done, unusual agencies began lending assistance. The World Bank mobilized $1.6 billion to finance the response and recovery, sending money directly to the governments of Liberia, Sierra Leone, and Guinea to plug budget gaps and pay for key supplies. The International Finance Corporation (IFC) made available $450 million in commercial financing to small and medium-size businesses; the IFC's business consultants gave advice to more than 800 businesses on health, security, and environmental efforts to help them recover.[5]

The United States Agency for International Development (USAID), which had received most of the money set aside by Congress to fight the outbreak, transitioned American dollars to rebuilding more fundamental elements of the economy. At the height of the crisis, as some countries banned flights and trade, food had become scarce. Markets closed, store shelves went bare. To prevent mass starvation, USAID's Food for Peace program delivered three hundred metric tons of rice to Liberia alone. Between the three West African nations, more than 1.5 million people received support from U.S. food programs. USAID also funded antidiscrimination campaigns aimed at eliminating any fears among the community about the thousands of survivors who had fought off the virus. Far from being a threat to their communities, their immune systems now swarmed with Ebola antibodies, which could help others who might contract the disease.

American governmental organizations like USAID and the Centers for Disease Control and Prevention (CDC) also went to work rebuilding the broken health-care system, including new immunization campaigns, maternal care, and, most basically, the rebuilding of trust between communities and health-care providers. The new message they aimed to spread: Ebola was no longer killing people, but avoiding health care for fear of catching Ebola would lead to other causes of death.

Though Ebola has been known to Western medicine for decades, the small scale of previous outbreaks meant few pharmaceutical companies had the incentive to spend money on researching and developing cures. The size and scope of the outbreak in West Africa changed that, and sent behemoth manufacturers scrambling for research.

The most well-known potential cure, ZMapp, was so difficult to produce that only thirty-six patients had ever received it. Eight of those patients died, but seven succumbed before the full course of the medicine could be delivered.

The drug, manufactured by a Kentucky-based company and derived from tobacco plants, won fast-track status from the U.S. Food and Drug Administration in September 2015. The full course of the drug sends particles that attach to the outside of the Ebola virus itself, neutralizing the virions while attracting killer immune cells. Scientists calculated a 91 percent probability that ZMapp could lead to a favorable outcome.[6]

A similar drug, dubbed MIL 77, underwent initial testing in China. Produced by Beijing Mabworks, the drug was used on British and Italian patients who survived. But it was so similar to ZMapp that the drug set off a fight between the American and Chinese governments over claims of patent infringements.

At least one more potential treatment, GS5734, showed early promise too. The drug quickly advanced from concept to phase one trials, then phase two trials by the summer of 2015. Travis Warren, the U.S. Army Medical Research Institute for Infectious Diseases (USAMRIID) scientist, called its progress "a phenomenal development time."

Others fell short.

The French National Institute of Health and Medical Research conducted trials of Favipirivir, a drug normally used to combat influenza viruses, for five months in Gueckedou, Guinea; Favipirivir showed promise among those with lower viral loads, but it did little to help those who were very sick.[7]

Developed by a company called Biocryst, BCX4430 showed promise inhibiting filoviruses in human cells and protected macaques from Marburg.[8] Amiodarone, a drug used to treat cardiac dysrhythmia, was tested on eighty patients in Sierra Leone through an Italian nongovernmental organization called Emergency. The tests were so poorly handled that fourteen British medical staffers stopped work at an Ebola treatment center in Freetown because they believed the drug would harm patients.[9]

Intravenous doses of TKM-130803 failed to improve conditions in a dozen patients in Port Loko. The manufacturer of brincidofovir tested its product in Monrovia, in a study led by Oxford University, and pulled out within a month when results went south.[10]

At the same time, scientists were working on a series of potential vaccines, which showed greater promise. Vaccines typically prime the body to recognize a foreign invader by infecting recipients with dead virus cells—as in influenza vaccines—or with a carrier virus that is not harmful to humans. Once the body's immune system is tipped off that viruses with certain proteins or structures must be attacked, the system will recognize a potentially harmful invader with a similar structure, like Ebola.

At the head of the pack was a drug with the maddeningly complicated name recombinant, replication-competent vesicular stomatitis virus-based vaccine expressing surface glycoprotein of Zaire Ebolavirus, or rVSV-ZEBOV for short.

Tests between April 1 and July 20, 2015, on 4,123 subjects in Conakry and eight other communities in Guinea showed a 100 percent efficacy rate after just a single injection. So did tests in Tonkolili and Bombali, in Sierra Leone. The vaccine, developed at USAMRIID and licensed to Merck Pharmaceuticals, created antibodies without inflicting any harm on humans.[11] In December 2016, scientists published their results in the *Lancet*, concluding that the vaccine had worked.[12] The U.S. Food and Drug Administration and the European Union fast-tracked the rVSV vaccine for approval, but even before it had cleared those hurdles public health officials had stockpiled 300,000 doses, in case of the next flare-up.

"While these compelling results come too late for those who lost their lives during West Africa's Ebola epidemic, they show that when the next Ebola outbreak hits, we will not be defenseless," said Marie-Paule Kieny, WHO's assistant director general and the lead author of the study, when the study was published.[13]

Another vaccine, replication-defective chimpanzee adenovirus 3 vector vaccine expressing Zaire Ebola virus glycoprotein—ChAd3-ZEBOV in the medical literature—served a similar function. The vaccine removes one protein from a chimp adenovirus, harmless to humans, and replaces it with a glycoprotein from the Ebola virus. That glycoprotein sticks out from the side of the virion, which gives the immune system an early warning, enabling it to recognize any foreign invader with a similar glycoprotein—that is, Ebola.[14]

The ChAd3 vaccine was given to 4,150 health-care workers in Mali, the United States, and Sierra Leone, to ensure that it is safe. The drug is in the process of advancing to phase-three testing. The only problem was it had to be stored at −80 degrees Celsius, a difficult prospect in the heat and humidity of equatorial Africa.

The number of vaccine and treatment candidates, and the promise they showed, gave global health officials reason to believe that the outbreak in West Africa would spawn a once-and-for-all cure for Ebola virus.

Speed, as in other areas of the outbreak response, was of the essence, and every day that a vaccine or a treatment was held up in trials was another day a patient in need was not getting drugs. But pharmaceutical companies are by nature cautious beasts, thanks to skittish legal departments, and the potential for exposing a global conglomerate to legal jeopardy tended to slow down the testing process.

GlaxoSmithKline, developing the ChAd3 vaccine candidate, told the Obama administration that it was particularly concerned about lawsuits. Any company that developed an Ebola vaccine would receive little in the way of profits; after all, the disease strikes only occasionally. A single lawsuit would wipe out those profits.

The White House turned to an obscure law for a solution: the Public Readiness and Emergency Preparedness (PREP) Act, passed after a swine flu vaccine made some recipients ill in 1976. The law allows the secretary of Health and Human Services to provide pharmaceutical companies with immunity from liability in tests of vaccines the government deems critical. Secretary Sylvia Burwell signed a PREP Act declaration covering vaccines in December 2014, and another covering proposed treatments in February 2015.

"We knew it would be a long time before we would really get any vaccine on any kind of widespread basis. So the question was, could you prevent these legal issues from getting in the way of the clinical trials,"

Ron Klain said later. GlaxoSmithKline had said it would not release its potential vaccine for clinical trials until it got immunity; the PREP Act declaration gave them an out.

Still, the American solution did not sit well with some in the global health community, and with others in West Africa. From the perspective of a poor African country, the United States had just given big multinational corporations an excuse to experiment on their citizens, and the country would have no legal recourse. That could give pharmaceutical giants unstated permission to circumvent some of their normal, careful procedures, and instead rush into the field with a drug candidate that could do more harm than good.

Gavi, the Global Vaccine Alliance, raised its own questions about the arrangement, which they feared would increase their costs, as drug makers demanded immunity from lawsuits relating to polio vaccines or other common treatments.

There were other public relations problems to consider as well. Glaxo-SmithKline researchers believed their vaccine would be 85 to 90 percent effective. From a public health standpoint, that rate of success would be high enough to ensure that an outbreak like Ebola would die out, for lack of unvaccinated hosts in which to live. But the 10 to 15 percent for whom the vaccine would not be effective would inevitably turn the blame back on the pharmaceutical company when they contracted the virus—potentially undermining the broader success of a vaccination campaign.

The biological facts of the Ebola virus were less important than the structural and societal reasons that an outbreak in a remote town had mushroomed into an international crisis—and very nearly a global catastrophe. In comprehensive case studies produced by everyone from the WHO to the CDC and smaller nongovernmental organizations, those who now turned their task toward preventing the next deadly disease identified seven main causes of Ebola's spread, and the solutions to those problems that would limit future outbreaks.

The causes, and their solutions, could be reasonably grouped into three broad categories: they were local, national, or international in nature.

At the local level, responders found three nations poorly equipped to provide access to basic services like water and sanitation. Second, tradition required family members to care for the ill and the dead, and West African funerary customs had undoubtedly helped the disease spread widely. The third cause was evident even to those who had never set foot in West Africa before Ebola descended like a fog—the lack of trust between local communities and their central governments in Conakry, Monrovia, and Freetown created an atmosphere in which the communities that most needed organized assistance were most reluctant to accept the help.

Nongovernmental organizations like Global Communities had spent years building proper sanitation and water service capacity. The villages that fully embraced the Global Communities Improved Water, Sanitation and Hygiene (IWASH) program, and therefore the connection between hygiene and health, experienced almost no Ebola cases. The Liberian environmental health technicians, who had helped those communities build their safer, more sanitary systems, then made up the burial teams who would enter villages and sit through long, drawn-out conversations explaining what Ebola was and what they were there to do to properly lay a victim to rest, without exposing other villagers. It was a message only Liberians could deliver to fellow Liberians, not one that westerners in their terrifying moon suits could convey. That led epidemiologists to conclude that a locally driven response, conducted by those who understood traditional customs and mores, helped break the virus's back. In some ways, a social science, anthropology, broke through what the hard sciences of biology and chemistry could not.

"We really broke through on some cultural practices," the National Security Council's Amy Pope recalled later. "We would now suggest that we should have anthropologists in any response."

Dan Martin, the CDC virologist who had been in the field in Sierra Leone, saw value in communicating a positive message. Early on, the World Health Organization and health ministries in all three countries tried to convey the danger of the Ebola virus by warning of its high fatality rate. That scared many who got sick, and convinced them to avoid the Ebola treatment units where they could receive treatment—and, more important, where they would be quarantined before they could infect family members and friends. Martin recalled:

Before this epidemic, most of us really thought of Ebola virus as, if you get Ebola, you're dead. You might as well say your prayers and do your will because you're on your way out. That was not an unreasonable thing for people to believe. . . . But one of the things that we saw, and we still don't have it fully nailed down on the science, but anecdotally we all know this to be the case, is that if we got people early on, when they first had their fever, when they first had their muscle aches, gave them oral rehydration solution, got them on IV, sustained their body so it didn't crash so badly during the dehydration and everything else of the disease, they actually stood a chance of fighting it off.

After initially scaring communities with messages about Ebola's dangers, the WHO later highlighted the growing number of survivors who returned home having beaten the disease. Those survivors proved that entering an Ebola treatment unit was not a death sentence.

"As we were able to get the message out that engaging with the system actually increases your chances for survival, that not only gave the community something to respond to, it gave us something to hang on to," Martin said. "We weren't just trying to keep people from taking somebody else with them while they died, we were actually trying to help these people get treatment so they could in fact recover."

At the national level, the weak public health systems in all three countries left their populations vulnerable to the spread of a deadly disease like Ebola, not to mention the more prevalent illnesses like Lassa, malaria, and cholera. Fragile infrastructure plagued responders trying to ferry supplies along rutted roads and into airports with bumpy tarmacs, while the lack of medical facilities meant that Liberia, Guinea, and Sierra Leone simply did not have enough space in which to safely treat Ebola patients.

"Lack of capacity made the Ebola virus chase us, more than we chased the Ebola virus," Tolbert Nyenswah told a conference at the Kaiser Family Foundation's headquarters in Washington in 2016.

Elements of the international response, from the CDC Foundation's purchase of hundreds of trucks and motorcycles to USAMRIID's laboratories and the rapid construction of Ebola treatment units, helped build that capacity. Military helicopters carrying blood samples from field hospitals to laboratories cut the diagnostic time from two or more days to a matter of just a few hours. So much capacity was added so quickly, first by Médecins Sans Frontières (MSF) and WHO, then by the U.S. military and other nongovernmental organizations, that some Ebola treatment units never admitted a single patient. By April 2015, only twenty-eight Ebola patients had been treated at two units built by the U.S. Army.[15]

As the world waits for the next major outbreak, the hodgepodge of national and international agreements covering vaccine and treatment clinical trials—and, more important, the gaps between those agreements—remain a significant and unaddressed challenge.

"We don't really have a global legal structure to deal with issues around that," Klain said.

Beyond drug treatments, governments and corporations used the Ebola outbreak to innovate in other areas, particularly in the types of equipment that health responders could use in the field.

The personal protection equipment that had been available worked, when used properly. But training responders to properly don and doff the bulky, cumbersome moon suits took days, and even some of the world's most experienced epidemiologists got it wrong. Both Tom Frieden from the CDC and Raj Shah from USAID were reprimanded when they missed steps in the safe doffing process.

"When you go in to treat a patient, you enter a hot zone. In that zone, you have to be fully clad: Gown, mask, gloves, double gloves, boot covers," Shah recalled. "Take 45 minutes in the zone, you're sweating, you have to pee, you're exhausted." Then the doffing profess begins, a twenty-step procedure as technicians spray the suit down with chlorine as each layer is removed.

To spur an easier system, the U.S. Global Development Lab brought together agencies and corporations from around the country. Steve Van-Roekel, who had served as the Obama administration's chief information officer, was dispatched to USAID to help coordinate efforts between NASA, Motorola, DuPont, and the Gates Foundation, among dozens of others, to come up with new equipment. The result was a special suit designed for treating patients in the field, outfitted with protected zippers and extra safety measures that reduced the safe doffing procedure from twenty minutes to thirty seconds.

Finally, on the international level, those evaluating the spread of Ebola cited the overcentralized nature of the World Health Organization, and the delays in international response caused by a bureaucratic behemoth that overestimated its own ability to respond to a crisis.

As the disease died down, officials from across the globe began taking a hard look at just what the response had gotten right, and more important, what agencies had gotten wrong. Virtually everyone, including the World Health Organization itself, pointed fingers at WHO. The agency had fallen flat in its ability to diagnose the severity of the Ebola outbreak, its ability to organize a global response, and even in its ability to offer assistance once it was on the ground. The United Nations Mission for Ebola Emergency Response (UNMEER) program, set up through the United Nations on the fly, had been such a disaster that American and other foreign officials frequently did not bother interacting with the rotating cast of uninformed and ill-prepared UN officials who parachuted in and out. The world, in short, needed a better answer for the next crisis.

Even before the outbreak was over, the first of several panels meant to assess the WHO's faults and failings came together. The WHO Ebola Interim Assessment Panel called the outbreak "a defining moment for the health to the global community," and it recommended wholesale changes at headquarters in Geneva.[16]

After months of review, the panel concluded that WHO had been woefully underfunded, and that it did not even have an emergency fund to pay for a fast response. Bureaucratic red tape meant it was impossible to place strong, independent directors in regional headquarters.

"WHO needs to be more operational, as distinct from normative. We're a really normative agency. In other words, we gather scientific evidence and provide advice on the nature of ill health," WHO's Chris Dye said in an interview. "We're not typically an operational agency. In other words, we don't do what the World Food Program does. We don't do what UNICEF does. We're not in the trenches."

The panel made six core recommendations. They suggested that the WHO enforce international health regulations that would spur countries to report outbreaks early, and to create a plan to build the capacity it would need to respond to any new epidemic. They wanted WHO to become more independent of its member nations, and to create a new threat level system that could respond to more minor outbreaks before they became epidemics.

Panel members also urged WHO to create disincentives against barriers to travel and trade in the event of an outbreak. Travel bans, like those proposed in the United States and implemented elsewhere, served only to isolate countries experiencing epidemics at a time when those countries needed help most. Had a travel ban been implemented in the United States, the thousands of doctors and technicians who streamed in to save lives would have been prevented from doing their work.

The panel also said that the United Nations secretary-general should make global health a priority of the Security Council. The UNMEER program had fundamentally erred, they said, in bypassing existing structures for health response instead of using the infrastructure that the United Nations already had at its disposal. The new agency had taken two months to set up, at a time when Liberia, Sierra Leone, and Guinea did not have two months to spare.

Most glaringly, the WHO panel turned its disapproving gaze to member states, which for decades had cut funding to Geneva. Even the United States was at fault—its funding had not kept up with the demands of an increasingly expensive, increasingly at-risk world.

"The member states need a lot of introspection, because the underlying problem is the way the member states have underfunded WHO," said Julio Frenk, a member of the panel. "When we analyze and criticize the WHO, for sure there's a lot to criticize of the secretariat, but there's also a lot to criticize of the members."

Some changes to WHO's internal structure have already taken place. Before the outbreak, one assistant director general had been in charge of humanitarian crises, and another had responsibilities overseeing outbreaks. Reflecting the increasingly interconnected nature of those two missions, the separate positions have now been merged into one. It is a seemingly minor change, but one that reflects the likely challenge that the next major outbreak will present.

Frenk, the president of the University of Miami who served as Mexico's secretary of health during the SARS (severe acute respiratory syndrome) outbreak, said that fixing WHO in time to address the next big crisis is a race against the clock. There have been diseases that are contagious but not deadly, and diseases that are deadly but not contagious.

"It's just a matter of time before we have the combination of a deadly and highly contagious micro-organism that is not localized to one part of the world. I worry we have not created the structures to deal with that," Frenk said. "If the world actually moves forward with these reforms, then we will be better prepared."

In West Africa, the new year brought sighs of relief. The worst of the Ebola outbreak was behind all three countries. The last week in which one hundred or more new cases were reported came in mid-March in Guinea and Liberia, and in April in Sierra Leone. Occasional fluctuations, caused by retroactive classifications, made the numbers jump around, and all three countries experienced minor outbreaks in the months to come. Guinea alone experienced ten minor "flares," as WHO termed them, between March and November 2015, but by December 29, the nation had gone forty-two days—two consecutive incubation periods—without a new case.

A month later, WHO declared an end to the outbreak in Liberia, after all known chains of transmission had been snuffed out. Liberia had experienced two flares since being declared Ebola-free in May. Sierra Leone was luckier; it had been disease-free since November.

But the end of one crisis left another intact. The public health systems in all three nations had been devastated, and the number of health-care workers left behind—even before the outbreak, inadequate to maintain public health—reached new lows. Facilities constructed by MSF, the CDC, and foreign militaries gave Guinea, Sierra Leone, and Liberia new infrastructure on which to build. Still, it will be years, perhaps decades, until all three countries rebuild the capacity to treat their own citizens, even without another outbreak.

The economic aftershocks will reverberate for years, as well. Lost commerce, tourism, and other economic activity likely cost the three nations $1.6 billion in 2015 alone, according to World Bank estimates.[17] Already three of the world's poorest nations, Liberia, Guinea, and Sierra Leone will take generations to recover from lost growth.

If officials in all three nations could take any solace, it was that the outbreak could have been much worse. The CDC's projections of up to 1.4 million people infected, which set off so much debate inside the U.S. administration, had been a worst-case scenario, but a possible scenario nonetheless. Those who had suffered gave the world the blueprint to defeat Ebola: better patient care guidelines, improved equipment, and a new sense of urgency in crafting a global epidemic response.

They also left behind gaping holes in West African society. From the tiny hillock on which Meliandou sits to the slums of Monrovia, Conakry, and Freetown, the final WHO report showed that 28,616 individuals had been stricken with the Ebola virus. Of those, 11,310 souls had perished.

TWENTY

The Next Outbreak

IN AUGUST 2016, I sat in the lobby of the Emory Conference Center Hotel, across the street from the Centers for Disease Control and Prevention (CDC) headquarters, nursing a glass of wine and preparing for a battery of interviews the following day, when I overheard a woman speaking about her experience fighting, and recovering from, the Ebola virus. It was Nancy Writebol, the Serving in Mission volunteer who had been infected two years previously. She had returned to Emory to address a group of young nurses, and to thank the medical professionals who had treated her during her darkest hours. For the brief few moments when I was fortunate enough to meet her, she offered a warm smile and a healthy handshake. She bore no outward scars that I could see.

But on the inside, Writebol and others have hinted at the lasting damage caused by a virus that haunts her, even though she has built up the antibodies necessary to make her immune. She has described in interviews with other reporters the pain she still experiences in her knees. Stairs are a problem. Nightmares haunt her at times.

Nancy Writebol, Kent Brantly, Craig Spencer, Nina Pham, Amber Vinson, and a handful of others who have not been named by those who cared for them are the American survivors of the largest outbreak of the most deadly disease known to man. Thousands of Liberians, Guineans, and Sierra Leoneans have survived as well, but their ordeals are not over. Even today, they struggle with the aftereffects of Ebola—the joint pain, the mental stress, the cultural stigma. The stress and strain of Ebola is so great that few want to discuss it. Writebol and Brantly did not respond to my repeated requests for interviews. After many e-mails back and forth, Spencer too declined to speak about his experience. He said he understood why the other two had not responded. More than a year later, the pain is too fresh.

I began reporting this story because the intersection between human society and the nature with which we interact is fascinating. Mankind's spread into the last remaining untouched parts of the natural ecosystem bears a cost—both to humans and to that ecosystem—with which neither side is prepared to deal. Conflict is inevitable; the outbreak of the Ebola virus in three desperately poor West African countries represents a worst-case scenario in microcosm.

What would—will?—happen when the next deadly pathogen with which we have no experience emerges? What would—will?—happen when someone infected with that pathogen boards an international airliner and winds up in the heart of London or New York or Beijing or Jakarta? I kept asking one question of those who had been so intimately involved in the response to the Ebola epidemic: Are we ready for the next one?

The answer, resoundingly, terrifyingly, is no.

Around the globe, the responders who are tasked with preventing or containing a viral epidemic are scrambling to evolve. Ebola exposed a woefully inadequate global health regime, one that proved to be in over its head almost from the beginning, thanks to years of bureaucratic bloat and international neglect. The World Health Organization (WHO) has engaged in a remarkable round of self-flagellation, consolidating some of its oversized bureaucracy and reforming itself to create a new directorate called the Health Emergencies Programme, established in 2016 with the explicit mission to deliver support to countries facing disasters, either natural or man-made.

WHO has made clear, too, that decades of stagnant appropriations from member nations, including the United States, have contributed to a budget crisis that has left what is ostensibly the world's frontline defense against deadly pathogens so weak that it is functionally unable to fulfill the role its member states expect. In her final months in office, Margaret Chan, WHO's director general, openly chastised member nations that have failed to deliver the money her agency needs.

"The problem can be succinctly stated," Chan told ambassadors at an October 31, 2016, meeting of donor nations in Geneva. "You expect a great deal from WHO. The organization is uniquely mandated to deliver. But someone must invest the requisite funds."

"The hard lessons from the Ebola outbreak underscore the need for WHO to have sufficient core capacity and readiness in place before the next crisis emerges. These are not capacities that can be built in the chaotic fray of a crisis," she said.

She was right.

In the absence of a competent and efficient WHO, the United States stepped in, deploying more responders to a public health crisis than ever before in the nation's history. More than 2,600 American troops spent weeks building Ebola treatment units, and more than 1,400 CDC employees swarmed the slums of big cities and the back roads of rural West Africa to track down as many victims as possible. Together with their Liberian, Guinean, and Sierra Leonean hosts, they built capacity to track, treat, and prevent a disease where none had existed.

During one of our interviews in his office just blocks from the White House, Ron Klain, the man who facilitated the U.S. government response to the crisis and whose nights were interrupted by constant false alarms about potential Ebola patients walking in to medical facilities across America, made a startling point about the American intervention: There aren't many other countries in the world where the United States could have done so much.

Though Liberia, Sierra Leone, and Guinea had suffered so much, the world had gotten lucky that the outbreak had occurred there, and not somewhere like the Middle East or Southeast Asia. The legacy of colonialism meant the United States, the United Kingdom, and to a lesser extent the government of France had the relationships, along with the money and the manpower, necessary to come to the aid of their close allies.

"We were able to divide the load between three Western countries. That's like a coalition-building fantasy game. That's never going to happen again," Klain said. "The disease broke out in one of a few countries on earth where the arrival of 3,000 U.S. troops was seen as a happy event, was seen as a blessed event."

"If this outbreak had been in Pakistan, or Indonesia? 'Good news, we're sending 3,000 troops from Fort Campbell, Kentucky, with guns.' No!" Klain said. "The most likely places where this is going to happen [next] are not places where you can send the 101st Airborne without fighting their way in."

The outbreak that claimed so many lives across international borders might have ended up like every other Ebola outbreak—a hot but brief-burning fire that ran out of fuel before it could spread—if Guinean and WHO officials had only recognized what they were looking at when they first arrived in Meliandou in December 2013. Indeed, at the same time the three West African nations were battling the virus, another outbreak struck the Democratic Republic of the Congo (DRC), in August 2014. The DRC has such a well-practiced Ebola response, given the myriad outbreaks that have taken place within its borders in the past three decades, that the virus never expanded beyond a few rural villages. Only sixty-six people contracted the virus, and forty-nine died.

But to stop a deadly outbreak, nations must have a competent and capable public health agency with four key elements: surveillance systems to identify an outbreak in its earliest stages, trained virus detectives to track down potential contacts, laboratory capacity to identify whatever is causing that outbreak, and rapid response teams capable of deploying in time to stop it from going any farther.

As it stands, the international community has had trouble agreeing on the very definitions countries use to evaluate their own health systems. Before the outbreak in West Africa, the hodgepodge of international consensus left it up to individual countries to evaluate their own health systems, and their ability to respond to deadly threats from natural pathogens, through a byzantine set of protocols and metrics that were virtually meaningless in their complexity. Now, a tool known as the Joint External Evaluation gives nations a common set of standards by which to judge their own capacity. The evaluation is voluntary, but it allows the international community to see potential blind spots that might otherwise have gone overlooked.

"We . . . have to convince the world that attention to the health infrastructure of their country is as important as anything else they do with their country," Anthony Fauci said.

Even before the extent of the Ebola outbreak was known, the Obama administration began pushing countries to join the Global Health Security Agenda, an international partnership that would put a premium on capacity building and a worldwide alarm system to sound warnings about the next killer virus that had undergone pilot programs in Uganda and Vietnam. Written into the supplemental spending bill Congress passed to curtail the outbreak were hundreds of millions of dollars aimed at bolstering that alarm system by funding new CDC-like agencies in dozens of countries.

But there are still nations that lack surveillance and detection capacity, which makes public health officials nervous. The global health chain is only as strong as its weakest link.

"We could get hit from one of those blind spots," Frieden said in one of our interviews. "So it's in our self-interest to close those blind spots."

Frieden's CDC has evolved tremendously in the wake of the outbreak in West Africa. An agency that was once proud of itself for deploying a dozen or so epidemiologists to fight a remote outbreak had sent more than 1,400 staffers to Liberia, Guinea, and Sierra Leone, tracked thousands of cases and tens of thousands of contacts, and trained an army of new health-care workers in all three countries.

In deploying so many staffers, the CDC also learned that the effects of an outbreak go beyond the effects of a virus. Frieden, who had been New York City's health commissioner in the aftermath of September 11, knew the potential dangers that mental health issues posed in the wake of such a traumatic experience. After the terror attacks, New York City had created a health registry that tracked 70,000 or so people who had been exposed to the dust and grit from the collapsing World Trade Center towers. While those who came down with respiratory issues had the most severe medical issues, their numbers were dwarfed by the thousands more who experienced crippling depression or posttraumatic stress disorder.

The same thing happened to those CDC staffers who came home from West Africa. "Even our most experienced people were really shaken by what they saw," Frieden said later.

Leisha Nolen had felt so lethargic when she returned from her first deployment, at the height of the outbreak. The CDC opened a special office dedicated to helping those who were coming back, offering counseling, time off, anything that would be necessary to a mental recovery. Hundreds of their employees took advantage of those offers. Dan Martin, who had worried about his friend John Redd's possible exposure, spoke out frequently about his decision to talk to a mental health professional, in hopes that his experience would help persuade others to seek out their own help.

"It took months to talk it out," Barry Fields, whose position running a lab at the ELWA hospital in Monrovia put him in close proximity with some of the sickest patients, said in August 2016. "I'm still talking it out."

But the epidemiologists, virologists, and laboratory technicians who had deployed from Atlanta came home with a deep sense of satisfaction. They had fought the most substantial outbreak in their lifetimes, one that could have become a global pandemic.

"We had been at the brink of an abyss, that it was absolutely possible that Ebola would get completely out of control and stay out of control for years," Frieden said. "We were able to avoid that catastrophe."

Perhaps most important, the CDC had, for the first time, developed a serious working relationship with the United States Agency for International Development Office of Foreign Disaster Assistance (USAID OFDA). Both Frieden and Jeremy Konyndyk, who headed the OFDA, had been surprised at the barriers built between the community of those who respond to natural and man-made disasters and the community of those who responded to outbreaks. They both thought that those barriers were false walls.

"An Ebola outbreak was not generally seen as something that would fall under the disaster response or humanitarian response community. The outbreak community was fairly distinct," Konyndyk said. "We need to do much more to bridge the divide globally between the emergency community and the outbreak community." The U.S. Congress is considering measures to establish a permanent bridge, through a Global Rapid Response Team.

The lessons that public health officials learned from the Ebola outbreak in West Africa have already been put into practice, the agencies responsible for responding to a viral outbreak already tested. Even before the final cases of Ebola were extinguished in West Africa, a new virus began appearing on international radars, one that spread far more easily than Ebola.

Like Ebola, the Zika virus was named for its geographic origin. The virus was first identified in the Zika Forest, a tiny strip of land along the Ugandan shores of Lake Victoria. Also like Ebola, Zika is not new—the first virologists to come across it had been on the hunt for Yellow Fever. They identified the Zika virus in a rhesus monkey in 1947.[1]

It is, in some ways, the opposite of Ebola. While scientists are still searching for the reservoir host that allows Ebola to lurk at the periphery of human existence, they know well where Zika resides, in *Aedes africanus* and *Aedes aegypti*, two of the most common mosquito species in the world. Though Zika poses little threat to healthy adults, the ubiquity of its reservoir host amplifies the potential to spread across the globe. Though Ebola is among the most deadly pathogens in the world, its relative lack of transmissibility hinders its ability to easily cause a global pandemic.

Zika broke out of central Africa first in 2007, when it showed up on the island of Yap in Micronesia. Micronesia is remote, but Brazil is not, and by 2015, WHO had reported the first series of cases in South America's most populous country. Within months, the virus had raced north, through Suriname, across the Panama Canal into El Salvador, Guatemala, and Mexico, and through the Caribbean islands of Martinique, Barbados, and Haiti.

On December 31, 2015, WHO reported its first case on American soil, on the island of Puerto Rico.

The staff inside any White House takes its direction from the tone and tenor set by the president they serve, and under President Obama, officials had maintained their cool during the Ebola outbreak, even when critics called them aloof and out of touch. But Obama had paid the political price for calm when Americans wanted evidence of decisive action, and he would not make the same mistake as Zika-plagued mosquitoes flew north.

"With Zika, we were out very early and very often from here," Amy Pope said in an interview in the ornate conference room inside the Eisenhower Executive Office Building once reserved for the secretary of war. "Then, we kind of took a back seat and we didn't see our role as publicizing what was happening on Ebola. . . . I think in hindsight our better course of action was to be more proactive. With Zika, here's what it is. Here's what we're requesting money for. Here's where our gaps are. And that's all in response to Ebola."

But even with more weapons in the arsenal, the global response has not stopped hundreds of children from suffering Zika's most horrific effects, like microcephaly, which causes infants to be born with underdeveloped brains. In the United States, Congress refused the Obama administration's requests to allocate billions of dollars to fight Zika, despite bipartisan support from Florida Senator Marco Rubio, a Republican whose state suffered the lion's share of infections on the mainland. Instead, Congress forced the White House to reallocate millions of dollars initially intended to fight Ebola, and to bolster the health systems both at home and abroad. Even after the Ebola scare, politics got in the way of the longer-term mission of building the global capacity to stop the next big outbreak.

What every epidemiologist, virologist, and public health expert agrees on is that the question the world faces is not whether the next big outbreak is coming, it is when. And mankind is sowing the seeds that will both speed the next outbreak and probably exacerbate its spread.

"You'll see other zoonotic diseases. I think you're going to see them more frequently. The idea that they're going to be, as they have been in the past, small and rural in nature is, in my view, unlikely. You just have a different level of urban integration and migration now, even in places like Asia and Africa," the former USAID director Rajiv Shah said.

Technological innovation beginning with jet aircraft has created a world in which almost anyone is only a plane connection away from the nearest hub airport, and from there only a handful of hours from New York or London or Beijing. A growing middle class in Africa, the Middle East, South America, and Asia means that more of us than ever have the financial ability to travel the globe.

At the same time, widespread poverty and the exploding human population means that we are living more densely than ever before and spreading our settlements farther into nature that has never contended with modern human civilization. In equatorial nations, slums abut wilderness, and the expansion of human settlements is decimating rainforests at a torrid pace. Human industrial activity is changing the global climate so much that tropical and subtropical zones are expanding north and south, away from the equator, which means mosquitoes and other creatures that could host new pathogens can now venture ever farther into newly habitable climate. The expansion of human civilization, an interconnected world, and a changing climate all conspire to pave the way for the spread of the fire of the next deadly pathogen.

Scientists fear that next pathogen will be some horrible combination of the worst traits of diseases like Ebola, Zika, and the common flu. A virus with the lethality of Ebola, carried by something as widespread as the common mosquito like Zika, and transmissible between humans like the flu is the stuff of Tom Frieden's nightmares.

"We always worry about flu. Flu is always the one that could do just terrible things, and that's something that we need to be continuously" vigilant about, Frieden said. "It spreads readily, and it kills a relatively high proportion of people if you get the wrong strain." He cited the Spanish influenza as our nearest comparison, a disease that infected as much as a quarter of the world's population during the early part of the twentieth century, killing 40 million people in the process.[2] Devastating though it was, that virus only killed about one in forty victims, or about 2.5 percent of those infected. Even something doubly as lethal, or less than a tenth as deadly as Ebola, would kill hundreds of millions of people today.

The next fire is coming, maybe from Kinshasa, maybe from Karachi, maybe from Kolkata or Kuala Lumpur or Kansas City. Someday in the future, it will leap from its host species into an unsuspecting human, who may then board a plane or infect a neighbor. As it spreads from Patient Zero, the global community will need to race back into the fire, identify the pathogen, identify a treatment and stop it before it spreads out of control.

The Ebola virus disease that ravaged Liberia, Guinea, and Sierra Leone was a devastating tragedy that claimed more than 11,000 lives, left three nations in ruins, and exposed a global health system left scrambling to stop its spread. If Ebola leaves a lasting legacy, Shah said, it should be as a wakeup call.

"There are so many much more scary pathogens out there," he said in his office overlooking Pennsylvania Avenue, just a block from the White House. "The world is still completely unprepared for it."

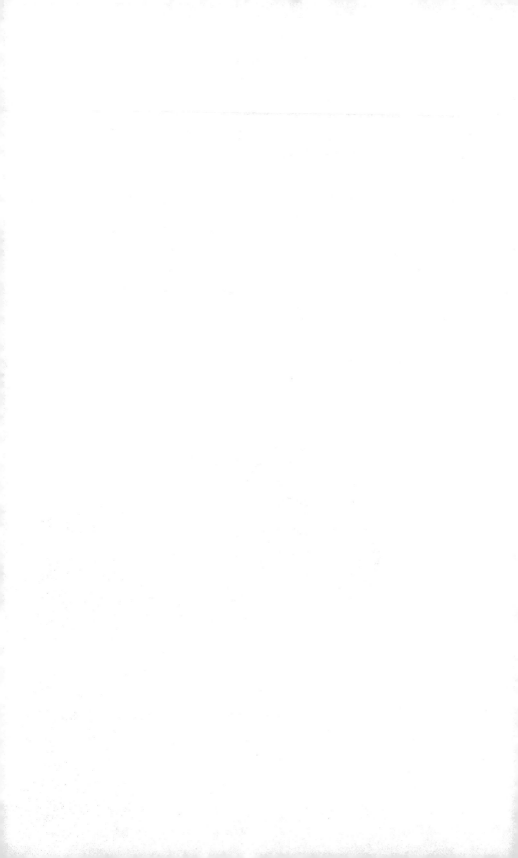

Acknowledgments

THIS BOOK WOULD NOT have been possible without the cooperation and support of dozens of people who worked to confront the Ebola outbreak, in Liberia, Guinea, and Sierra Leone, in Geneva at the World Health Organization (WHO), at the White House, the Centers for Disease Control and Prevention (CDC), National Institutes of Health (NIH), and the U.S. Army Medical Research Institute for Infectious Diseases (USAMRIID). My thanks go to all of them, including—but not limited to—Ron Klain, Anthony Fauci, Tom Frieden, Amy Pope, Gayle Smith, Rajiv Shah, Jeremy Konyndyk, Randy Schoepp, Robert Garry, Senator Chris Coons, Fabian Leendertz, Chris Dye, Julio Frenk, Lieutenant Colonel Ross Lightsey, Colonel Brian Gentile, Captain Jeff Kugelman, and Major General Gary Volesky. I was fortunate enough to speak with Hans Rosling, the Swedish physician and statistician, several months before he passed away in February 2017.

Among the dozens of U.S.-based nongovernmental organizations that mobilized to fight the outbreak, three were particularly generous with their time: the CDC Foundation, and its former president Charlie Stokes; Global Communities, where Piet deVries and Brett Sedgewick sat for long interviews; and World Vision, and the unfailingly gracious David Robinson.

At the CDC, Leisha Nolan, Barry Fields, Peter Kilmarx, John Brooks, David Blackley, Joe Woodring, Kimberly Lindblade, Dan Martin, John Redd, and Blanche Collins endured hours of questions. Benjamin Haynes, Erin Sykes, and Mansi Das helped set up interviews and graciously dealt with a thousand fact-check requests. At USAMRIID, Caree Vander Linden organized an eye-opening visit to Fort Detrick, where Colonel Gentile, Schoepp, Captain Kugelman, David Norwood, Travis Warren, and others patiently explained the science. Captain Michael Schmoyer of the U.S. Public Health Service donated his time as well. At the White House, Peter Boogaard, Ned Price, and Eric Schultz helped with background and arranging interviews. Max Gleischman, who accompanied UN Ambassador Samantha Power on her trip to West Africa, provided insights into the international response at the United Nations. Lieutenant Colonel Lightsey spent hours on the phone answering questions.

I leaned heavily on contemporaneous on-the-ground reporting from journalists including Joshua Hammer, who documented the heartbreaking final days of Sheik Umar Khan; Richard Preston, writing in the *New Yorker*; Bryan Burrough, who reported in *Vanity Fair* on the response to the outbreak in Dallas; Norimitsu Onishi, who reported from the ground for months for the *New York Times*; and others. WHO, Médecins Sans Frontières, and the CDC all documented their own work, much of which I used to give the fullest possible picture. Preston himself may have planted the seeds of this book two decades ago with his own book, *The Hot Zone*, and the subsequent movie version, *Outbreak*, which I still remember seeing in middle school. I was inspired by authors whose books have covered previous outbreaks, including Laurie Garrett's *The Coming Plague*, and David Quammen's *Spillover*.

At Brookings Institution Press, my thanks to editorial director William Finan and managing editor Janet Walker for their interest in this story, and for dealing with a nervous first-time author who probably sent them too many drafts. I'm grateful to my colleague Ashley Perks, design director at *The Hill*, who designed the beautiful map of Liberia, Guinea, and Sierra Leone. Matthew Carnicelli, of Carnicelli Literary Management, provided valuable guidance as this book came into being.

And thanks, as well, to the mentors who have shepherded my career in journalism: Chuck Todd, who gave me my first job and trusted me to help his own book project; Bob Cusack; Steven Ginsberg; and too many more to count. Cynthia Wilson, my mother, taught me how to write as I grew up. Bart Wilson, my father, struck the delicate balance between encouraging me and offering constructive criticism. My wonderful wife Veronica didn't let me give up when my writing struggled, and our son Max, who joined us as this book was being finalized, is an incredible gift.

There is no way to compile the stories of the thousands of people, Liberians, Sierra Leoneans, Guineans, Americans, Brits, and French, who raced toward the fire when others ran away, or to tell the stories of the more than 28,000 people who fell victim to Ebola, and the holes left behind by the 11,000 who died. One can hope that the vaccine finalized in late 2016 will mean there are no more stories of future Ebola outbreaks to tell.

I am incredibly grateful to all who participated in this project.

Notes

Chapter 1

1. Almudena Mari Saéz and others, "Investigating the Zoonotic Origin of the West Africa Ebola Epidemic," *EMBO Molecular Medicine* 7, no. 1 (January 2015), pp. 17–23.

2. Sylvain Baize and others, "Emergence of Zaire Ebola Virus Disease in Guinea," *New England Journal of Medicine* 371 (2014), pp. 1418–25; Saéz and others, "Investigating the Zoonotic Origin."

3. Jeffrey E. Stern, "Hell in the Hot Zone," *Vanity Fair*, September 11, 2014 (www.vanityfair.com/news/2014/10/ebola-virus-epidemic-containment).

4. See Centers for Disease Control and Prevention, "Lassa Fever" (www.cdc.gov/vhf/lassa/).

5. Stern, "Hell in the Hot Zone."

6. Pierre Formenty, "Ebola Diaries: First signals—March 2014" (www.who.int/features/2015/ebola-diaries-formenty/en/).

7. Kevin Sack and others, "How Ebola Roared Back," *New York Times*, December 30, 2014.

8. Ibid.

9. Formenty, "Ebola Diaries."

10. Sack and others, "How Ebola Roared Back."

11. Stern, "Hell in the Hot Zone."

Chapter 2

1. David Quammen, *Spillover: Animal Infections and the Next Human Pandemic* (New York: Norton, 2012).

2. Thucydides, *History of the Peloponnesian War*, book 2, chapter 7.

3. Laurie Garrett, *The Coming Plague: Newly Emerging Diseases in a World Out of Balance* (New York: Farrar, Straus and Giroux, 1994).

4. For an in-depth history of Ebola outbreaks, see Quammen, *Spillover*.

5. Jeffrey Taubenberger, "The Origin and Virulence of the 1918 'Spanish' Influenza Virus," *Proceedings of the American Philosophical Society* 150 (March 2006), pp. 86–112.

6. Quammen, *Spillover*.

7. Garrett, *The Coming Plague*, p. 123.

8. World Bank, OECD statistics (http://data.worldbank.org/indicator/NY.GDP .MKTP.CD http://data.worldbank.org/indicator/SP.DYN.LE00.IN?view=chart).

Chapter 3

1. Rob Fowler, "Ebola Diaries: Fighting an Uphill Battle," World Health Organization, April 2014 (www.who.int/features/2015/ebola-diaries-fowler/en/).

2. Stéphane Hugonnet, "Hitting the Ground Running," World Health Organization, March 2015 (www.who.int/features/2015/ebola-diaries-hugonnet/en/).

3. Jeffrey Stern, "Hell in the Hot Zone," *Vanity Fair*, September 11, 2014.

4. Quoted in "'Ebola Not in Liberia,'" *Liberian Observer*, March 27, 2014.

5. Quoted in ibid.

6. Stern, "Hell in the Hot Zone."

7. Quoted in "Liberia Needs US$1.2M to Contain Ebola," *Liberian Observer*, March 28, 2014.

8. Fowler, "Ebola Diaries."

9. "How Ebola Roared Back," *New York Times*, December 29, 2014.

10. Cristiana Salvi, "Ebola Diaries: Regaining the People's Trust," World Health Organization, April 2014 (www.who.int/features/2015/ebola-diaries-salvi/en/).

Chapter 4

1. As posted on Twitter @HaertlG, April 1, 2014 (https://twitter.com/HaertlG /status/451023126185672704).

2. "How Ebola Roared Back," *New York Times*, December 29, 2014.

3. Ibid.

4. Lisa George, "CDC Steps Up Response to Ebola Outbreak in West Africa," August 13, 2014 (http://news.wabe.org/post/cdc-steps-response-ebola-outbreak-west -africa).

5. "How Ebola Roared Back."

6. Ibid.

7. Ibid.

8. Richard Preston, "Inside the Ebola Wars," *New Yorker*, October 27, 2014.

Chapter 5

1. "How Ebola Roared Back," *New York Times*, December 29, 2014.

2. Helene Sandbu Ryeng, "Harisson Sakilla: Liberia's First Ebola Survivor," medium.com, April 15, 2015 (https://medium.com/ebola-stories/harisson-sakilla -liberia-s-first-ebola-survivor-881309013a61).

3. Richard Preston, "Inside the Ebola Wars," *New Yorker*, October 27, 2014.

4. Madeline Drexler, "On The Ground: Alumnus Battles the Nightmare in Liberia," *Harvard Public Health Magazine*, December 16, 2014 (www.hsph.harvard .edu/magazine/magazine_article/the-ebola-response/).

Chapter 6

1. Joshua Hammer, "My Nurses Are Dead and I Don't Know If I'm Already Infected," medium.com, January 12, 2015 (https://medium.com/matter/did-sierra -leones-hero-doctor-have-to-die-1c1de004941e).

2. Quoted in "Interview: Sierra Leone's Ebola Doctor Feared for His Life," *Politico SL*, May 8, 2014 (http://freemediasl.com/articles/interview-sierra-leones -ebola-doctor-feared-his-life).

3. Erika Check Hayden, "Infectious Disease: Ebola's Lost Ward," *Nature*, September 24, 2014.

4. Ibid.

5. Quoted in "Interview: Sierra Leone's Ebola Doctor."

6. Hayden, "Infectious Disease."

7. Denise Grady and Sheri Fink, "Tracing Ebola's Outbreak to an African 2-Year-Old," *New York Times*, August 10, 2014.

8. Hayden, "Infectious Disease."

9. Hammer, "My Nurses Are Dead."

10. Ibid.

11. Ibid.

Chapter 7

1. Folasade Ogunsola, "How Nigeria Beat the Ebola Virus in Three Months," theconversation.com, May 13, 2015 (http://theconversation.com/how-nigeria-beat -the-ebola-virus-in-three-months-41372).

2. World Health Organization, "Nigeria Is Now Free of Ebola Virus Trans-mission," press release, October 20, 2014 (http://who.int/mediacentre/news/ebola /20-october-2014/en/).

3. Michael Daly, "How Bureaucrats Let Ebola Spread to Nigeria," DailyBeast .com, August 14, 2014.

4. Ibid.

5. Katherine Harmon Courage, "How Did Nigeria Quash Its Ebola Outbreak So Quickly?" *Scientific American*, October 18, 2014.

6. Daly, "How Bureaucrats Let Ebola Spread."

7. Will Ross, "Ebola Crisis: How Nigeria's Dr. Adadevoh Fought the Virus," BBC News, October 20, 2014 (www.bbc.com/news/world-africa-29696011).

8. Courage, "How Did Nigeria Quash Its Ebola Outbreak?"

9. F. O. Fasina and others, "Transmission Dynamics and Control of Ebola Virus Disease Outbreak in Nigeria, July to September 2014," *Eurosurveillance* 19, no. 4 (October 9, 2014) (http://eurosurveillance.org/images/dynamic/EE/V19N40 /art20920.pdf).

10. Daly, "How Bureaucrats Let Ebola Spread."

11. Courage, "How Did Nigeria Quash Its Ebola Outbreak?"

12. Fasina and others, "Transmission Dynamics and Control of Ebola Virus."

Chapter 8

1. Lisa Abbott, "Notable Alumni: Dr. Kent Brantly," Heritage Christian School (www.heritagechristian.net/discover/notable-alumnni/post/~board/notable -alumni/post/kent-brantly).

2. Brenda Goodman, "The Race to Save Dr. Brantly: The Inside Story," WebMD.com, September 12, 2014 (www.webmd.com/a-to-z-guides/news/20140912 /saving-kent-brantly#1).

3. "Ebola Survivor Nancy Writebol: All Doctors Could Say Was 'We Are So Sorry,'" NBC News, September 3, 2014 (www.nbcnews.com/storyline/ebola -virus-outbreak/ebola-survivor-nancy-writebol-all-doctors-could-say-was-we -n194361).

4. Alexandra Zavis, "Ebola Doctor's Dilemma: Two Patients, and Drugs Enough for One," *Los Angeles Times*, December 24, 2014.

5. Goodman, "The Race to Save Dr. Brantly."

6. Richard Preston, "Inside the Ebola Wars," *New Yorker*, October 27, 2014.

7. Zavis, "Ebola Doctor's Dilemma."

8. Ibid.

9. Goodman, "The Race to Save Dr. Brantly."

10. Preston, "Inside the Ebola Wars."

11. Zavis, "Ebola Doctor's Dilemma."

12. "Ebola Survivor Nancy Writebol."

13. Zavis, "Ebola Doctor's Dilemma."

14. Martin Enserink, "How Two U.S. Patients Changed the Debate about Using Untested Ebola Drugs," *Science*, August 7, 2014 (www.sciencemag.org /news/2014/08/how-two-us-patients-changed-debate-about-using-untested-ebola -drugs).

15. World Health Organization, "WHO to Convene Ethical Review of Experimental Treatment for Ebola," press release, August 6, 2014 (www.who.int /mediacentre/news/statements/2014/ethical-review-ebola/en/).

16. Enserinak, "How Two U.S. Patients Changed the Debate."

Chapter 9

1. Madeline Drexler, "On The Ground: Alumnus Battles the Nightmare in Liberia," *Harvard Public Health Magazine*, winter 2015 issue (www.hsph.harvard .edu/magazine/magazine_article/the-ebola-response/).

2. Alexandra Zavis and Christine Mai-Duc, "Clashes Erupt as Liberia Seals Off Slum to Prevent Spread of Ebola," *Los Angeles Times*, Aug. 20, 2014 (www .latimes.com/world/africa/la-fg-africa-liberia-ebola-quarantine-curfew-20140820 -story.html).

3. Normitsu Onishi, "As Ebola Grips Liberia's Capital, a Quarantine Sows Social Chaos," *New York Times*, p. A1, August. 29, 2014 (www.nytimes.com /2014/08/29/world/africa/in-liberias-capital-an-ebola-outbreak-like-no-other .html).

4. Ibid.

5. Norimitsu Onishi, "Quarantine for Ebola Lifted in Liberia Slum," *New York Times*, p. A4, August. 30, 2014 (https://www.nytimes.com/2014/08/30/world /africa/quarantine-for-ebola-lifted-in-liberia-slum.html).

6. World Health Organization, "Ebola in Liberia: Misery and Despair Tempered by Some Good Reasons for Hope" (www.who.int/csr/disease/ebola/ebola-6 -months/liberia/en/).

7. Médecins Sans Frontières, "Liberia: MSF's New Ebola Management Centres Already Overwhelmed," press release, August 27, 2014 (www.msf.org /article/liberia-msf's-new-ebola-management-centres-already-overwhelmed).

Chapter 10

1. Mark Anderson, "Ebola: Airlines Cancel More Flights to Affected Countries," *The Guardian*, August 22, 2014.

2. Norimitsu Onishi, "In Liberia, Home Deaths Spread Circle of Ebola Contagion," *New York Times*, September 25, 2014.

3. Michael Osterholm, "What We're Afraid to Say about Ebola," *New York Times*, September 12, 2014.

Chapter 11

1. Brady Dennis, "CDC 'Disease Detective' Talks about Challenges of Fighting Spread of Ebola Virus," *Washington Post*, August 1, 2014.

2. Kai Kupferschmidt, "Star Statistician Hans Rosling Takes on Ebola," *Science Magazine*, December 2, 2014.

Chapter 12

1. Ross Lightsey, "Fighting Ebola: An Interagency Collaboration Paradigm," *Joint Forces Quarterly* 81 (March 29, 2016).

2. United Nations, "With Spread of Ebola Outpacing Response, Security Council Adopts Resolution 2177 (2014) Urging Immediate Action, End to Isolation of Affected States," press release, September 18, 2014 (www.un.org/press/en/2014/sc11566.doc.htm).

3. Barbara Starr, "Army Major General Speaks to CNN from inside Ebola Quarantine," CNN, October 28, 2014 (www.cnn.com/2014/10/28/politics/starr-ebola-general-interview/index.html).

Chapter 13

1. Avi Selk, "Ebola Victim Came to Dallas to Realize His U.S. Dreams," *Dallas Morning News*, October 6, 2014.

2. Bryan Burrough, "Ebola in the U.S.," *Vanity Fair*, February 2015.

3. Selk, "Ebola Victim Came to Dallas."

4. Dianna Hunt and Claire Cardona, "Hospital Had Made Preparations for Treating an Ebola Case," *Dallas Morning News*, September 30, 2014.

5. Burrough, "Ebola in the U.S."

6. Ibid.

7. Ibid.

8. Ibid.

9. Tawnell Hobbs and Paige Kerley, "Student Who Had Contact with Ebola Patient Attended Dallas School Despite Request," *Dallas Morning News*, October 2, 2014.

10. Avi Selk, "Among Those Closest to Dallas Ebola Case, Confusion Reigns," *Dallas Morning News*, October 2, 2014.

11. Burrough, "Ebola in the U.S."

12. Ibid.

13. Dianna Hunt and Sherry Jacobson, "Dallas Hospital under Fire as Accounts of Ebola Patient's Initial Release Change," *Dallas Morning News*, October 4, 2014.

14. "Record Details Thomas Eric Duncan's Last Days," Associated Press, October 11, 2014 (www.oregonlive.com/today/index.ssf/2014/10/thomas_eric_duncans_final_days.html).

15. Burrough, "Ebola in the U.S."

16. Dan Morse, "Nina Pham, Nurse Who Contracted Ebola, Is Now Free of Virus and Leaves NIH," *Washington Post*, October 24, 2014.

17. Burrough, "Ebola in the U.S."

18. Alan Blinder, "Amber Joy Vinson, Dallas Nurse Treated for Ebola, Is Released from Hospital," *New York Times*, October 28, 2014.

Chapter 15

1. Michael Osterholm, "What We're Afraid to Say about Ebola," *New York Times*, September 12, 2014.

2. Craig Spencer, "Having and Fighting Ebola: Public Health Lessons from a Clinician Turned Patient," *New England Journal of Medicine* 372 (March 19, 2015), pp. 1089–91 (www.nejm.org/doi/full/10.1056/NEJMp1501355).

3. Tom Frieden, the head of the Centers for Disease Control and Prevention, had spent seven years running New York City's health department before President Obama tapped him for the job in Atlanta.

4. "Kaci Hickox, Maine Nurse Who Defied Quarantine, Details Ebola Mission," video, *Bangor Daily News*, January 6, 2015 (http://bangordailynews.com/2015/01/06/health/kaci-hickox-maine-nurse-who-defied-quarantine-speaks-out-about-ebola-mission/).

5. Anemona Hartocollis and Emma Fitzsimmons, "Tested Negative for Ebola, Nurse Criticizes Her Quarantine," *New York Times*, October 26, 2014.

6. Naheed Rajwani, "UTA Grad Isolated at New Jersey Hospital as Part of Ebola Quarantine," *Dallas Morning News*, October 25, 2014.

7. Sara Fischer, "Christie's Office: Quarantined Woman Headed to Maine," CNN, October 27, 2014 (www.cnn.com/2014/10/26/politics/ebola-quarantine-christie-white-house/index.html).

8. Sarah Dutton, Jennifer De Pinto, and others, "Do Americans Believe There Should Be a Quarantine to Deal with Ebola?" CBS News, October 29, 2014 (www.cbsnews.com/news/do-americans-believe-there-should-be-a-quarantine-to-deal-with-ebola/).

9. Monmouth University, "NJ: Gov. Christie Gets High Marks on Ebola," Monmouth University Poll, November 6, 2014 (www.monmouth.edu/assets/0/3221 2254770/32212254991/32212254992/32212254994/32212254995/40802189893/fd 2f1e6ea751402a849adccc57a30ec5.pdf).

Chapter 17

1. Norimitsu Onishi, "In Liberia, Home Deaths Spread Circle of Ebola Contagion," *New York Times*, September 25, 2014.

2. Kevin Sack and others, "How Ebola Roared Back," *New York Times*, December 29, 2014.

3. Alice Urban, "A Year of Response: Liberia Country Director Piet deVries Reflects on Global Communities' Fight Against Ebola," Global Communities, March 12, 2015 (www.globalcommunities.org/node/38063).

4. Onishi, "In Liberia, Home Deaths Spread."

5. Lucy Draper, "Frontline Health Workers Were Sidelined in $3.3bn Fight Against Ebola," *Newsweek*, May 19, 2015 (www.newsweek.com/ebolasierra-leone liberiaguineawest-africawhoworld-health-organisation-604666).

6. Ibid.

Chapter 18

1. Lucy Draper, "Frontline Health Workers Were Sidelined in $3.3bn Fight Against Ebola," *Newsweek*, May 19, 2015.

2. Centers for Disease Control and Prevention, "Outbreaks Chronology: Ebola Virus Disease" (www.cdc.gov/vhf/ebola/outbreaks/history/chronology.html#modalId String_outbreaks).

3. Norimitsu Onishi, "Empty Ebola Clinics in Liberia Are Seen as Misstep in U.S. Relief Effort," *New York Times*, April 12, 2015.

4. For Obama's full remarks, see "Remarks by the President on America's Leadership in the Ebola Fight," White House, Office of the Press Secretary, February 11, 2015 (https://obamawhitehouse.archives.gov/the-press-office/2015/02/11 /remarks-president-americas-leadership-ebola-fight).

Chapter 19

1. Seema Yasmin, "Why Ebola Survivors Struggle with New Symptoms," *Scientific American*, February 29, 2016 (www.scientificamerican.com/article/why -ebola-survivors-struggle-with-new-symptoms/).

2. Jim Wappes, "Studies on Ebola Survivors Show Range of Complications," Center for Infectious Disease Research and Policy, University of Minnesota, February 25, 2016 (www.cidrap.umn.edu/news-perspective/2016/02/studies-ebola -survivors-show-range-complications).

3. "Recovering from the Ebola Crisis," report issued by the United Nations, World Bank, European Union, and the African Development Bank (http://www .undp.org/content/undp/en/home/librarypage/crisis-prevention-and-recovery /recovering-from-the-ebola-crisis---full-report.html).

4. Robbie Corey-Boulet, "Oxfam: $1.9B in Ebola Aid Not Delivered by Donors," Associated Press, January 31, 2016 (www.sltrib.com/home/3482655-155/oxfam -19b-in-ebola-aid-not).

5. World Bank, "World Bank Group Ebola Response Fact Sheet," brief, April 6, 2016 (www.worldbank.org/en/topic/health/brief/world-bank-group-ebola-fact-sheet).

6. Richard Davey and others, "A Randomized, Controlled Trial of ZMapp for Ebola Virus Infection," *New England Journal of Medicine* 375 (October 13, 2016), pp. 1448–56 (http://www.nejm.org/doi/full/10.1056/NEJMoa1604330).

7. Daouda Sissoko and others, "Experimental Treatment with Favipiravir for Ebola Virus Disease (the JIKI Trial): A Historically Controlled, Single-Arm Proof-of-Concept Trial in Guinea," *PLOS Medicine*, March 1, 2016 (http://journals.plos .org/plosmedicine/article?id=10.1371/journal.pmed.1001967).

8. Travis Warren and others, "Protection against Filovirus Diseases by a Novel Broad-Spectrum Nucleoside Analogue BCX4430," *Nature* 508 (April 17, 2014), pp. 402–5 (www.nature.com/nature/journal/v508/n7496/full/nature13027 .html).

9. Sarah Boseley, "Untested Ebola Drug Given to Patients in Sierra Leone Causes UK Walkout," *The Guardian*, December 22, 2014 (www.theguardian.com /world/2014/dec/22/ebola-untested-drug-patients-sierra-leone-uk-staff-leave).

10. Robert Roos, "Trial Suggests Potential for Sequential Use of 2 Ebola Vaccines," Center for Infectious Disease Research and Policy, University of Minnesota, April 20, 2016 (www.cidrap.umn.edu/news-perspective/2016/04/trial-suggests -potential-sequential-use-2-ebola-vaccines).

11. Ana Maria Henao-Restrepo and others, "Efficacy and Effectiveness of an rVSV-vectored Vaccine Expressing Ebola Surface Glycoprotein: Interim Results from the Guinea Ring Vaccination Cluster-randomised Trial," *Lancet*, July 31, 2015 (www.thelancet.com/pb/assets/raw/Lancet/pdfs/S0140673615611175.pdf).

12. Ana Maria Henao-Restrepo and others, "Efficacy and Effectiveness of an rVSV-vectored Vaccine in Preventing Ebola Virus Disease: Final Results from the Guinea Ring Vaccination, Open-label, Cluster-randomised Trial (Ebola Ca Sufit!)," *Lancet*, December 22, 2016 (www.thelancet.com/journals/lancet/article /PIIS0140-6736(16)32621-6/fulltext).

13. World Health Organization, "Final Trial Results Confirm Ebola Vaccine Provides High Protection against Disease," press release, December 23, 2016 (www.who.int/mediacentre/news/releases/2016/ebola-vaccine-results/en/).

14. Milagritos Tapia and others, "Use of ChAd3-EBO-Z Ebola Virus Vaccine in Malian and US Adults, and Boosting of Malian Adults with MVA-BN-Filo," *Lancet Infectious Diseases* 16, no. 1 (January 2016), pp. 31–42.

15. Norimitsu Onishi, "Empty Ebola Clinics in Liberia Are Seen as Misstep in U.S. Relief Effort," *New York Times*, April 12, 2015.

16. World Health Organization, "Report of the Ebola Interim Assessment Panel" (www.who.int/csr/resources/publications/ebola/report-by-panel.pdf).

17. World Bank, "Ebola: Most African Countries Avoid Major Economic Loss but Impact on Guinea, Liberia, Sierra Leone Remains Crippling," press release, January 20, 2015 (www.worldbank.org/en/news/press-release/2015/01/20/ebola-most -african-countries-avoid-major-economic-loss-but-impact-on-guinea-liberia -sierra-leone-remains-crippling).

Chapter 20

1. Veronica Sikka and others, "The Emergence of Zika Virus as a Global Health Security Threat," *Journal of Global Infectious Diseases* 8, no. 1 (February 11, 2016), pp. 3–15.

2. Jeffrey Taubenberger and David Morens, "1918 Influenza: The Mother of All Pandemics," *Emerging Infectious Diseases* 12, no. 1 (January 2006), pp. 15–22 (wwwnc.cdc.gov/eid/article/12/1/05-0979_article).

Index